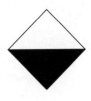 # Psychology and health promotion

Health Psychology

Series editors:
Sheila Payne and Sandra Horn

Published titles

Psychology and Health Promotion
Paul Bennett and Simon Murphy

Pain: Theory, Research and Intervention
Sandra Horn and Marcus Munafo

Psychology and health promotion

Paul Bennett and Simon Murphy

Open University Press
Buckingham • Philadelphia

Open University Press
Celtic Court
22 Ballmoor
Buckingham
MK18 1XW

and
1900 Frost Road, Suite 101
Bristol, PA 19007, USA

First Published 1997

A catalogue record of this book is available from the British Library

ISBN 0 335 19766 3 (hb)   0 335 19765 5 (pb)

Library of Congress Cataloging-in-Publication Data
Bennett, Paul, 1956–
    Psychology and health promotion / Paul Bennett and Simon Murphy.
       p.   cm.
    Includes bibliographical references and index.
    ISBN 0-335-19766-3 (hardcover). – ISBN 0-335-19765-5 (pbk.)
    1. Clinical health psychology.   2. Health promotion—Psychological
aspects.   I. Murphy. Simon, 1963– .   II. Title.
    R726.7.B46   1997
    613–dc21   97-9042
                                                                          CIP

Typeset by Graphicraft Typesetters Limited, Hong Kong
Printed in Great Britain by Biddles Ltd, Guildford and King's Lynn

Contents

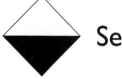 Series editors' foreword

This new series of books in health psychology is designed to support post-graduate and postqualification studies in psychology, nursing, medicine and paramedical sciences, as well as the establishment of health psychology within the undergraduate psychology curriculum. Health psychology is growing rapidly as a field of study. Concerned as it is with the application of psychological theories and models in the promotion and maintenance of health, and the individual and interpersonal aspects of adaptive behaviour in illness and disability, health psychology has a wide remit and a potentially important role to play in the future.

In this book, Bennett and Murphy have moved beyond medical and educational models of health promotion to introduce psychological theories. They make few assumptions about the level of psychological or health knowledge of readers. Psychosocial and cognitive mediators of health are defined in the early chapters, and followed by detailed consideration of how individual lifestyle changes can be facilitated. There is also an introduction to population level health promotion interventions aimed at reducing the incidence of conditions such as heart disease, HIV/AIDS and some cancers. This broadens the traditional psychological approach, with its emphasis on individual differences, and includes consideration of environmental influences such as workplace and housing. It also draws on sociological constructs such as ethnicity and socio-economic status as mediators of health. The book ends with some challenging ideas and highlights possible research agendas and practical applications for health promotion.

Sheila Payne and Sandra Horn

Introduction:
why psychology?

Health promotion is concerned with enhancing health and preventing disease. Since its inception, its primary focus has been on the prevention of physical disorders such as coronary heart disease and cancer. Only more recently, has health promotion moved towards issues of mental health. Why then, have psychological theory and methods become integral to much health promotion? Is this not the province of public health physicians and educationalists? This text will attempt to answer these questions. We do so first by giving some consideration to what we mean by health promotion and how psychology may facilitate its goals.

Approaches to health promotion

The primary focus of health education has been to change individual behaviour, or intrapersonal factors such as attitudes and beliefs thought to mediate behaviour, in order to promote better health. Tonnes (1990: 2), for example, defined health education as 'any planned activity which promotes health or illness related learning; that is, some relatively permanent change in an individual's competence or disposition'. An American perspective is provided by Green and Iverson (1982), who defined it as 'any combination of learning experiences designed to facilitate voluntary adoptions of behaviour conducive to health' (1982: 2).

In contrast, the historical development of health promotion has seen a move beyond education to include economic, environmental, social and legislative measures to enhance population health. Green and Iverson (1982), for example, define health promotion as 'any combination of health education and related organizational, economic and environmental supports for behavior conducive to health' (1982: 321).

Underlying these definitions are two very different perspectives on health: social regulationist and radical structuralist (Caplan 1993). The social regulation approach accepts that existing structures support and regulate society and that change can be effected within these structures. In this model, health education is primarily focused on modifying individual cognitions and providing the behavioural skills necessary for health-behaviour change. In contrast, the radical structuralist approach states that ill-health is a product of unequal power in society, which results in conflict, tension and inequalities, including those of health. From this perspective, health promotion should be concerned with fundamental change in the way society is organized and how its resources are distributed. This could be achieved, for example, by raising public awareness of issues and community and political activism. A radical structuralist approach to health promotion warns of the dangers of victim blaming (Ryan 1976; Crawford 1977) considered inherent within a health education approach.

In defence of a health educationalist perspective, Tonnes (1990: 5–6) states

> it is rather ingenuous to believe that all health problems might be solved through social policy. There are many occasions when individuals need personal understanding, skills and support. It is therefore more realistic to define victim blaming as the process of ignoring social structural factors while focusing exclusively on the individual.

It is also apparent that empowering individuals can also lead to political or social activism on their part and that facilitating political and social change requires an understanding of the individuals within those structures. Accordingly, we argue that psychology has a role to play in programmes aimed at both individual and social or environmental change, providing guiding theory for both health education and promotion and radical structuralist and social regulation approaches.

The layout of the book

Health promotion draws on many disciplines and knowledge bases to inform its practice. To compare the extent of each discipline's contribution may be invidious. Nevertheless, it is generally acknowledged that psychological theory and practice can contribute substantially to the practice of health promotion and psychological theory has provided a strong basis for the development and implementation of some of the most important programmes of population-based health promotion so far conducted (Bunton and MacDonald 1992). However, much health promotion remains atheoretical or uses inappropriate psychological theory (Bunton *et al.* 1991). This may result, at least in part, from a lack of texts integrating psychological theory with health promotion practice. This text attempts to do exactly this. It is divided into four parts.

Part I: Mediators of health and health behaviours

The first part of the book has two chapters. Chapter 1 adopts both a regulationist and structuralist view of risk factors for disease. It begins by reviewing the evidence linking a number of risk behaviours to disease. It then considers how societal processes may contribute to the disease process, and considers how psychological processes may contribute to differentials in morbidity and mortality associated with gender, socio-economic status and ethnicity. Finally, it considers the link between stress and health. Chapter 2 involves a more considered review of some of the factors which determine the uptake and maintenance of health behaviours. It describes and critiques a number of social cognitive models, identifying internal processes thought to guide health-related behaviour.

Part II: Facilitating individual change

Health promotion works at a number of levels. Some initiatives are targeted at individuals; some at entire populations. Part II considers how behavioural change may be facilitated through work at an individual or group level. Chapter 3 describes some of the theory of individual work. It examines strategies of change through the provision of verbal or written information, motivational interviewing, and more complex counselling. The latter focuses particularly on Egan's model of problem-focused counselling. The chapter ends with a detailed consideration of the application of Egan's model, combined with specific additional components, in the context of smoking cessation and stress management. Chapter 4 then examines how effective such interventions have been in practice, drawing on research from both primary and secondary prevention settings and with a variety of behavioural change end-points.

Part III: Facilitating population change

While much psychological theory has been developed to explain individual behaviour, its theories still have strong applicability to population-based attempts at behavioural change. Accordingly, three chapters are devoted to linking psychological theory and population level health promotion initiatives. Chapter 5 examines how psychological principles may inform social, environmental, and legislative attempts at engendering behavioural change and improving health. In the next chapter we introduce a number of theories informing the use of mass communication and consider their effectiveness in changing attitudes and behaviour. Chapter 7 then describes some of the more important population-based programmes, including those targeted at whole city populations and the worksite, which have used many of the principles examined in isolation in the previous chapters.

Part IV: What next?

This part comprises only one chapter, yet we feel this is a particularly important one. So far, the book has adopted a model of orthodox mainstream psychology and considered its value with scant regard for the individual in the context within which they live. Here, we explore a number of social and other environmental processes which influence the behaviour and health of the individual, focusing in particular on symbolic interactionism (Blumer 1969). We finally call for health promotion to improve the quality of life of individuals, not merely reduce their risk of disease, and consider how this may be achieved.

The book is a brief review of an extensive, and expanding, literature. Each chapter could be extended to fill one or more books. We have therefore had to present issues briefly, using examples of relevant research rather than providing complete area reviews. We hope you enjoy what you read and become interested in reading further on some topics. To assist you in this, we provide a list of suggested reading at the end of each chapter.

Suggested reading

Bunton, R. and MacDonald, G. (1992) Health promotion: discipline or disciplines? In R. Bunton and G. MacDonald (eds) *Health Promotion: Disciplines and Diversity.* London: Routledge.

Ewles, L. and Simnett, I. (1995) *Promoting Health: A practical guide.* (3rd edn) London: Sucarti Press.

Naidoo, J. and Wills, J. (1994) *Health Promotion: Foundations for Practice.* London: Bailliere Tindall.

Tonnes, K. and Tilford, S. (1994) *Health Education: Effectiveness, Efficiency and Equity.* (2nd edn) London: Chapman Hall.

Mediators of health and health behaviours

Psychosocial mediators of health

Health promotion is premised on the understanding that the behaviours in which we engage and the circumstances in which we live impact on our health, and that appropriate changes will improve health. Traditionally, the focus of health education programmes has been on modifying health-related behaviours such as smoking and exercise. Perhaps reflecting a paradigm shift towards more structuralist approaches, more recent consideration has been given to the importance of social and environmental variables in mediating health (WHO 1991). A third strand of research has investigated the impact of psychological factors such as stress and personality on health status.

Of course, this neat delineation into separate influences on health presents a false simplicity. Health outcomes of relevance to health promotion are the result of a complex interaction between biological, social, environmental, and psychological factors. Social class may influence health, at least in part, as a consequence of an unequal distribution of life opportunities and stress throughout society (Carroll *et al.* 1993), work stress is associated with increased smoking rates (Ames and Janes 1987), poor access to leisure facilities may reduce uptake of exercise programmes (Lee and Owen 1985), and so on. Nevertheless, this chapter addresses each of these issues in turn. It first examines the relationship between lifestyle and health before adopting a structuralist perspective and examining how social and environmental variables may impact on our health. The final section examines some of the processes through which environmental stressors and stressed responses may influence health. As this is a psychology text, the opportunity is taken to examine some of the processes underlying the latter in more detail.

Lifestyle and health

About 50 per cent of premature deaths in western countries can be attributable to lifestyle (Hamburg *et al.* 1982). Smokers, on average, reduce their life expectancy by five years, individuals who lead a sedentary lifestyle by two to three years, and so on. Four behaviours in particular are associated with disease: smoking, alcohol misuse, poor nutrition and low levels of exercise – the so-called 'holy four' (McQueen 1987). Conversely, rarely eating between meals, sleeping for seven to eight hours each night, and eating breakfast nearly every day have been associated with good health and longevity (Breslow and Enstrom 1980). More recently, high risk sexual activity has been added to the risk factor list.

Dietary habits

Evidence from nearly half a million people attests to the role of blood cholesterol levels as a major risk factor for coronary heart disease (CHD; Law *et al.* 1994). The MRFIT study (Stamler *et al.* 1986), for example, followed over 350,000 adults for six years and found a linear relationship between blood cholesterol level and the incidence of CHD or stroke. The risk for individuals within the top third of cholesterol levels was three and a half times greater than those in the lowest third. These data have been replicated in numerous studies, and the risk for CHD attributable to blood cholesterol is unchallenged.

Cholesterol combines with lipoproteins at differing stages of its metabolism within the body, to form high density and low density lipoprotein (HDL and LDL) cholesterol; HDL is considered the 'good' cholesterol as it is involved in transportation from the arteries and other tissues to the liver, LDL is considered the 'bad' cholesterol because it contributes to the formation of plaque within the arteries. Although the ratio between LDL and HDL cholesterol may differ both between individuals and in the same individual over time, measures of total cholesterol provide a reasonable measure of risk. While there is no threshold level below which there is no risk for CHD, risk is significantly increased by cholesterol levels above 5.2 mmol/litre for those aged over 30 years, and of 4.7 mmol/litre for younger people (Leon 1995). These margins place about two-thirds of the UK population at some risk for CHD (Lewis *et al.* 1986).

Blood cholesterol levels are to a significant degree mediated by dietary intake of fats. With this in mind, appropriate levels of fat consumption have been established in a number of countries. These are typically substantially below the population norms. In the USA, for example, approximately 44 per cent of calories are consumed as fat (USBC 1989), contrasting with the recommended levels of 30 per cent (USDHHS 1988). Even these levels are considered high for those identified as being at particular risk for CHD. Ornish *et al.* (1990), for example, advocated that only between 10 and 20 per cent of calories should be consumed as fat by this population. Raised blood cholesterol levels, equivalent to those mediated by inappropriate diet, may also be consequent to a stress-induced failure to metabolize cholesterol in the liver (Ornish *et al.* 1990). In addition, cholesterol levels may be mediated by exercise levels (Kannel 1995) and genetic factors (Steinberg 1979).

Diet is also linked to cancer. Austoker (1994), for example, suggested that up to 25 per cent of cancer-related deaths are attributable to dietary factors, including high fat, low fibre and inadequate vitamin and mineral intake. At present, it is not possible to formulate a precise definition of which cancers are causally related to diet and what proportion of them are due to specific dietary components. However, a number have been identified as risk or protective factors. Risk factors include meat, total fat, saturated fat, preserved food and salt. Protective factors include fruit, vegetables, fibre, anti-oxidants, fish oils and calcium (Austoker 1994). Interestingly, smokers may reduce their risk of developing lung cancer if their diet includes high levels of anti-oxidants found in fruit and vegetables. Conversely, a low intake of fruit and vegetables combined with high alcohol intake significantly increases risk for oral, pharyngeal and oesophageal cancers (WHO 1990).

Smoking

The adverse health consequences of smoking are widely acknowledged. It is considered responsible for 25 per cent of all CHD-related deaths, 80 per cent of cases of chronic obstructive airways disease, and 90 per cent of deaths associated with lung cancer, as well as contributing to the development of cancers of the larynx, mouth, oesophagus, pancreas and bladder (Smith and Jacobson 1988).

The health consequences of smoking become evident over relatively long periods of time, and present morbidity levels reflect changes in smoking which occurred up to three decades ago. Increased lung cancer rates in women over the last two decades are thought to be a consequence of the rapid increase in the numbers of women smoking during and after the Second World War. In contrast, reductions in lung cancer rates among men are not thought to result from any behavioural change. Rather, they reflect changes in the composition of cigarettes during the post-war years (Smith and Jacobson 1988). Reductions in ingested tar of over 50 per cent, following the introduction of filters to cigarettes, are thought to contribute to reductions in cancer levels, but have not impacted on those for CHD. Smoking not only affects the smoker; about 25 per cent of lung cancers that occur in non-smokers are considered to be attributable to passive smoking (Wald *et al.* 1986).

In the west, smokers are now a minority in every age and social group. In the UK, for example, adult smoking rates between 1976 and 1986 fell by 24 per cent in men and 18 per cent in women, to 35 and 31 per cent of the population respectively (Smith and Jacobson 1988). Only among young women are smoking rates actually rising (Goddard and Ikin 1988). Differentials in smoking levels are also found according to socio-economic status, with the economically advantaged smoking less than those occupying the lower socio-economic groups. However, those individuals in the higher socio-economic groups who do smoke cigarettes may be more vulnerable to their adverse health effects than those who are more economically deprived (Hein *et al.* 1992; see below).

Excessive alcohol consumption

Excessive alcohol consumption may impact adversely on both short and long-term health. Up to 40,000 people in the UK are thought to die prematurely as a consequence of excess alcohol intake (Royal College of General Practitioners 1986). Although cirrhosis of the liver is the disease most frequently associated with alcohol damage, most deaths result from cancer (Anderson *et al.* 1993); three per cent of all cancers are attributable to excess alcohol. Even more dramatically, a combination of smoking and high alcohol consumption results in a 44-fold increase in oesophageal cancer (Smith and Jacobson 1988). The negative consequences of excess alcohol intake are not just medical, but involve social and psychological outcomes. Twenty per cent of psychiatric admissions, 60 per cent of parasuicides, 30 per cent of divorces, and 40 per cent of incidences of domestic violence are associated to some degree with alcohol misuse (Royal College of Psychiatrists 1986).

The relationship between consumption and harm does not appear to be linear in all cases. Risk for heart disease is now thought to be lowered by moderate consumption of alcohol (e.g. Hennekens *et al.* 1978), mediated by increased HDL cholesterol levels in such drinkers (see Leon 1995). However, a linear relationship between physical harm and alcohol consumption is found for all other outcomes including cirrhosis, cancer and stroke (Anderson *et al.* 1993).

Defining what is meant by excess alcohol consumption has proven far from simple. As this text is being written, UK government guidelines for what is considered 'sensible drinking' are being revised from a recommendation of 21 units or less for men, and 14 units or less for women, per week to 28 and 21 units respectively (Department of Health 1995). However, the appropriateness of changing these guidelines in the absence of new evidence has been strongly challenged (see the *British Medical Journal*, vol. 293), and a number of health promotion agencies and alcohol agencies have been reluctant to adopt these guidelines. Accordingly, there remains a lack of clear advice concerning the recommended limits to consumption. Most evidence presently available is based on 'sensible' limits of 21 units per week for men and 14 units for women. Using these criteria over a quarter of men and 10 per cent of women presently drink beyond the recommended limits in the UK (Thomas *et al.* 1992).

Exercise

Those who are physically active throughout their adult life live longer than those who are sedentary. Paffenbarger *et al.* (1986), for example, monitored leisure-time activity in a cohort of Harvard graduates for a period of 16 years. Those who expended more than 2,000 kcal of energy in active leisure activities per week lived, on average, two and a half years longer than those classified as inactive. Exercise is protective against both CHD and some cancers (Blair et al. 1986). How this protection is achieved, whether through short intense periods of exercise (Simons-Morton et al. 1988) or longer, more frequent less intense periods (Blair et al. 1986) appears irrelevant and no additional health gain is achieved by exceeding these limits.

About a quarter of the UK population engage in health promoting levels of exercise, with a similar picture in the USA (Ivancevitch and Matteson 1989). Recent years have also seen dramatically increased levels of exercise participation. In Wales, for example, data from the 1985 Heartbeat Wales Survey suggested that only one in five men and 2 per cent of women took sufficient exercise to protect them from CHD (Directorate of the Welsh Heart Programme 1986). By 1990, 27 per cent of the population engaged in this level of exercise (Norman et al. in press).

Participation rates differ according to age, sex, and socio-economic factors. Those who engage in exercise are more likely to be young, male and well-educated adults, members of higher socio-economic groups, and those who have exercised in the past. Those least likely to exercise tend to be in the lower socio-economic groups, older individuals, and those whose health is likely to be at risk as a consequence of being overweight and smoking cigarettes (Dishman 1982). Obstacles to exercise include not having enough time, lack of support from family or friends and perceived incapacity due to ageing (Dishman 1982; Sallis and Hovell 1990).

High risk sexual behaviour

By the beginning of 1992, nearly 2,500,000 people had died of AIDS worldwide, and 19,500,000 were known to be HIV positive (Mann et al. 1992). UK figures indicate a marked increase in the prevalence of other sexually transmitted diseases and unwanted pregnancies (Friedman 1989; Catchpole 1992) – evidence of the high prevalence of unsafe sex practices (see below) and perhaps heralding future increases of HIV infection and AIDS. In contrast to the previous demographics of the disease, adolescent heterosexuals form an increasingly at-risk group for AIDS, accounting for about 20 per cent of all newly reported cases in the USA (Stiff et al. 1990). Within this group, young women and ethnic minorities appear to be at particular risk. Joseph (1988), for example, highlighted findings that AIDS-related illnesses form the leading cause of death for young women aged 25 to 34 in the USA and the third leading cause for those between 15 and 19 years old. Ethnic minority adolescents, the majority of whom were poor urban blacks, accounted for 53 per cent of new AIDS cases (Buttrose 1987). A similar picture is emerging in the UK. Although the majority of newly diagnosed cases of AIDS are still gay and bisexual men, the incidence of new cases among this group is falling slowly as the incidence of such cases among the heterosexual community rises more rapidly (Day 1996).

Clearly, adolescent sexual behaviour places many at high risk for disease. They are a sexually active group. Findings from a British survey (HMSO 1987), for example, revealed that nearly half the adolescents aged between 16 and 17 have had at least one sexual partner during the previous year. However, they are unlikely to plan intercourse (Friedman 1989), and only half use any form of contraception (Cubis et al. 1985). In a well-educated sample of heterosexual students, Hawkins, et al. (1995) reported that the most frequent 'safer sex' behaviour was the use of the contraceptive pill. The least frequent sexual practice, reported by only 24 per cent of the sample, was the use of condoms or dental dams.

Such inappropriate behaviour may stem from a lack of knowledge (Chapman and Hodgson 1988). However, even high levels of knowledge may not be associated with engaging in safer sex practices (Valdisseri et al. 1988; Allard 1989). Perhaps a more important factor is that a majority of young persons do not see themselves as at risk of HIV infection (NCHS 1988) or have feelings of invulnerability towards the disease (Greig and Raphael 1989).

Social and environmental influences on health

There is substantial evidence that behaviour influences health status. What is also becoming increasingly evident is that the place we occupy in society also impacts substantially on our health; indeed, such factors may overwhelm the impact of individual behaviours. In the next section, we summarize some of the evidence linking gender, socio-economic status (SES), and ethnicity to health and consider some of the mechanisms through which these associations may be mediated. We return to these issues in the final chapter, where we consider the implications of these links for the practice of health promotion.

Gender and health

Women, on average, live longer than men. In the UK, between 1984 and 1987, the average life expectancy for men was 71 years; that of women, 77 years (United Nations 1990). Paradoxically, men assess their health more positively, report fewer symptoms of illness, contact physicians less frequently and experience less acute non-life threatening illnesses than women (Reddy et al. 1992).

Most explanations for these differences have focused on biological factors. Oestrogen probably protects women against coronary heart disease, through reducing clotting tendency and reducing blood cholesterol levels, while testosterone may serve to increase platelet aggregation (McGill and Stern 1979).

Men may also have a greater, and more pathogenic, physiological response to environmental stressors, exhibiting greater stress hormone, blood pressure and LDL cholesterol rises to laboratory stressors than women (Matthews and Stoney 1988). However gender differences may not necessarily implicate genetic differences. Work by Lundberg *et al.* (1981), for example, has shown that women in traditionally male occupations exhibit the same level of stress hormones as do men in similar jobs. These findings suggest that at least some of these differences may be driven by social and cultural processes, not hardwired biological processes.

Gender specific societal processes may also influence the health behaviour of individuals. The relative power accorded to different genders, for example, may powerfully influence the negotiation of sexual intercourse and sexual behaviour. Abbott (1988) reported that 38 per cent of an Australian sample of young women reported having intercourse when they did not want it. Similarly, a number of British studies have found that young women are disempowered in sexual negotiations such that their intentions to engage in safer sex practices are not translated into action (Holland *et al.* 1990; Abraham *et al.* 1995). A further example of the impact of societal mores on health-related behaviour can be found in studies of participation in exercise and fitness programmes. Here, low participation rates for women are frequently ascribed to family responsibilities and joint work–home responsibilities and the societal norms which support such behavioural choices (Green *et al.* 1986).

Whatever the cause, men behave differently to women. Men are more likely to be overweight, smoke more frequently using higher nicotine and tar cigarettes, eat less healthily, and drink more heavily than women (Reddy *et al.* 1992). They are also more likely to encounter adverse working conditions, and contact with carcinogens and accidents. The former may work synergistically with health habits to contribute to greater levels of early mortality.

Together, these data suggest that while biological factors may mediate some of the differentials in health status between men and women, others are behaviourally or societally mediated. Gender differential in life expectancy may arise, to a significant degree, from the cumulative effects of different social worlds that men and women experience from the moment of their birth. Consequently, the health status of both men and women can be improved by modifying societal conditions that promote health-damaging behaviours.

Socio-economic status and health

Health varies markedly with SES, both for measures of all-cause mortality and all major diseases (Marmot *et al.* 1991). These differences are progressive, and throughout the social classes. They hold for women as well as men (Arber 1989) and are characteristic of all western countries studied (Wilkinson 1992).

A number of theories have been proposed to explain this relationship. First, variations in health may reflect differences in lifestyle. However, while those in the more deprived social groups do engage in more health damaging behaviours such as smoking or drinking excessively, this does not fully explain the health–SES relationship. In the 10-year long follow-up of the Whitehall 1 study (Marmot *et al.* 1984), when variations in smoking, obesity, plasma cholesterol and blood pressure were statistically partialled out of the risk equation, occupational status-related differentials in health still remained. Corroborative evidence emerged from a 17-year prospective study of CHD in Danish men (Hein *et al.* 1992). Adjusting for age, blood pressure, body mass index and alcohol consumption, men who smoked evidenced a risk for CHD 3.5 times that of non-smokers. However, when these data were analysed according to class, white-collar smokers evidenced a risk ratio of 6.5:1 in comparison to non-smokers. Among blue-collar workers, no additional risk for CHD was conferred by smoking status. Fewer middle-class people may smoke, but paradoxically, those that do may be particularly vulnerable to the health-damaging effects of smoking. Conversely, the impact of smoking on the health of the lower SES participants was overwhelmed by social factors.

A second explanation for these health differentials is that people in lower socio-economic groups may be exposed to more environmental insults, including industrial toxins (Hunter 1955), low quality and damp accommodation (Martin *et al.* 1987), and air pollution levels (Watt and Ecob 1992). While these could be used to explain the differentials, two factors militate against this conclusion. First, the available data suggest that socio-economic health gradients persist into the materially better-off strata; that is, health stratification is not simply a matter of the most deprived in society suffering exceedingly poor health. Second, the differentials remain when comparisons are made within populations which share the same working environment (Marmot *et al.* 1984). Accordingly, while poverty and environmental factors contribute to disease, they do not fully explain the socio-economic health differentials.

Comparisons of life expectancy across different western countries, however, provide some further clues as to the nature of this relationship. These show life expectancy not to be determined by the absolute wealth of the society and the individuals within it. Rather, the distribution of wealth within a society is substantially predictive. The narrower the distribution, whatever its absolute level, the better the overall health of the nation. Accordingly, although Japan and Cuba differ substantially on measures of economic wealth, both have relatively equitable distributions of income and long life expectancies throughout their populations (Wilkinson 1992). It seems that for the majority of people in western countries, health hinges on relative perhaps more than absolute living standards. These data have led a number of commentators (Wilkinson 1992; Carroll *et al.* 1993) to conclude that the environment and standard of living impact on our health not only through physical causes but also through social and psychological processes as well.

Psychological explanations for health inequalities have received scant consideration, and any explanation must at present remain speculative. However, three interrelated psychological processes appear implicated. Stress is unequally distributed through society, and those in the lower socio-economic groups report more stressors, including everyday hassles, than individuals in higher groups (Myers *et al.* 1974). In addition, the less well-off have less control over their environment and personal resources to mediate the impact of such stressors (Sleutjes 1990). Third, social support, a powerful mediator of health status, is less available to individuals in the lower socio-economic groups (Adler *et al.* 1994). Each of these factors has been implicated in the development of disease; attention has yet to be given to their role within a socio-economic framework. However, even if these mediating factors can be identified and modified in some individuals, reducing the health burden attributable to differentials in socio-economic status may still depend on reducing the inequalities themselves (Carroll *et al.* 1996).

Ethnicity and health

Data from the USA identifies a strong association between ethnicity and health status. Blacks have higher age-adjusted mortality rates for heart disease, cancer, liver diseases, diabetes and pneumonia than whites. They are also much more likely to die from violence (Markides 1983). In the UK, rates of ill-health and mortality amongst ethnic minorities differ from those of the white population, but there are also marked differences between them. Data from the 1991 census (see Balarajan and Raleigh 1993), for example, revealed rates for CHD among men from the Indian subcontinent to be 36 per cent higher than the national average, and 46 per cent higher for women. These differences were greatest for those aged between 20 and 39 years, where members of this group evidenced rates of CHD two to three times higher that for whites. For African-Caribbeans, excess mortality was associated with strokes and hypertension. Among this group, the incidence of strokes in men was 76 per cent higher than the national average, and 110 per cent higher in women. Mortality related to hypertension was four times greater than the national average in males and seven times greater in females. Mortality rates associated with cancer among Asians and African-Caribbeans have been lower than the national average, although they are now rising (Barker and Baker 1990).

Differences in health behaviour are associated with both race and gender. In the USA, black females drink less alcohol and smoke less cigarettes than white females, while males resemble their white counterparts (Gottlieb and Green 1987). In the UK, the prevalence of smoking is uniformly low across women from all ethnic groups but differs across groups for men (Balarajan and Yuen 1986; Waterson and Murray-Lyon 1989). Alcohol-related morbidity is high among Asian males of Punjabi origin and African-Caribbean men (Cochrane and Bal 1989; Clarke *et al.* 1990), while a high dietary fat intake and an increasing incidence of diabetes have been observed among Asians (McKeigue *et al.* 1985; Fox and Shapiro 1988). The influence of ethnicity on health behaviour is perhaps highlighted when examining transmission of HIV. The most common exposure route for whites is through sexual intercourse between men; for blacks it is through heterosexual intercourse, while for Asians it is mixture of both (Calman 1991).

A structuralist explanation for these health differentials is also relevant. Ethnicity is frequently confounded with class, with a significant proportion of members of ethnic minorities occupying lower SES groups. Accordingly, factors which increase morbidity for disease among these groups will also affect many of the members of ethnic minorities (Goldberg and Comstock 1980; Robinson 1984). In addition, ethnic minorities may experience wider sources of stress as a consequence of discrimination and racial harassment, and experience more problems in gaining access to health services such as cancer screening and antenatal care than their white counterparts (Doyle 1991; Narang and Murphy 1994).

Stress and health

Stress is not a unitary construct. It is a process involving a complex interaction between environmental, psychological and physiological processes. Much of the research investigating the relationship between stress and health has examined the effect of these variables in isolation from one another, or has differed in its theoretical conceptualization of stress. Accordingly, to establish the relationship between stress and health it is necessary first to define stress, and to work from this definition to examine its relationship to health and disease.

Stress as a physiological process

At a fundamental level, the relationship between stress, health and disease status is mediated by physiological processes. These primarily involve the two divisions of the autonomic nervous system: the sympathetic and the parasympathetic. They arise from the medulla oblongata in the brain stem, and enervate and control the functioning of most of the internal organs, including the heart, arteries, skeletal muscles, and colon. The sympathetic system is involved in arousal, while the parasympathetic system is involved in calming or reducing arousal. At times of stress, activation of the sympathetic system is predominant, at times of relaxation, the parasympathetic. Because these systems are mediated by neurotransmitters, collectively known as catecholamines, their activation is extremely fast, but is not sustained.

More prolonged activation results from hormonal processes. Activation of the sympathetic nervous system results in the medulla (or centre) area of the adrenal glands, situated above the kidneys, releasing the neurotransmitter hormones epinephrine and norepinephrine. These enter the bloodstream and reach the organs controlled by the sympathetic system to maintain longer periods of activation. At the same time, a second 'stress' system is activated. This involves sympathetic activation of the pituitary gland, situated under the hypothalamus in the brain, which releases a number of hormones, including adrenocorticotrophic hormone (ACTH). In turn, ACTH stimulates the adrenal cortex to release hormones known as corticosteroids. These increase availability of energy stores of fats and carbohydrates, helping maintain arousal. They also inhibit inflammation of damaged tissue.

One of the first coherent explanatory models of the association between stress and health (Selye 1956) suggested that this sympathetically mediated activation is a non-specific response to all stressors, whatever their nature, involving three stages: alarm (driven primarily by sympathetic processes), resistance (mediated by hormonal changes), and exhaustion. This final stage occurs when adaptive reserves are depleted through repeated or long-term stressful encounters. It is a stage at which resistance is no longer possible and disease onset may occur. Withdrawal from the stressor as a consequence of disease permits a period of regeneration and recovery. Consistent overactivation of the sympathetic nervous system may contribute to the development of a number of chronic diseases, including coronary heart disease, skin disorders, diabetes, and a number of gastro-intestinal disorders (e.g. Bennett 1995).

The exact aetiology of each disease process may differ. In the case of heart disease, for example, episodes of high sympathetic arousal consequent to stress are associated with the release of fatty acids into the bloodstream. If these are not completely utilized during the period of stress through, for example, high levels of physical activity, they are metabolized by the liver into cholesterol. This is then deposited as atheroma within the arteries. In addition, short-term increases in blood pressure at the time of sympathetic activation may damage the atheroma already within the arteries, leading to the initiation of repair processes, further exacerbating the development of atheroma.

At some point, a clot may be torn off a damaged artery wall, perhaps during an episode of increased blood pressure. If this reaches the arteries of the heart or brain and is too large to pass through an artery, it will occlude the artery and prevent blood flow beyond, resulting in a heart attack (myocardial infarction or MI) or stroke. Catecholamines released during the stress process may also affect blood viscosity directly (Markovitz and Matthews 1991), making the platelets more likely to clot, and increasing risk of an acute vascular event. Because persistent high sympathetic arousal also inhibits activation of the immune system, long-term stress may increase risk for immunologically mediated diseases such as viral infections (Cohen et al. 1991) or exacerbate the development of some cancers (Levy and Schain 1987; Levy *et al.* 1988).

Life events as sources of stress

In contrast to Selye's physiological model of stress, Holmes and Rahe (1967) adopted a psychological model of stress, disregarding the physiological processes. They explored the relationship between major life events and the development of disease. In this, they considered similar life events to carry the same degree of stress to all individuals and constructed a hierarchy of stressors, with scores varying from 0 to 100 (Holmes and Rahe 1967), with higher scores reflecting more highly stressful events. Their theory stated that the higher an individual's score on this hierarchy, the more likely they were to experience a stress-related disease. A number of studies have used this paradigm, and found some evidence of a modest association between the occurrence of life events and accidents and illness (see Cohen 1979).

However, the notion of an invariant hierarchy of stress has a number of problems. In particular, the scale does not take into account the meaning or impact of an event for the individual. For example, the score for the most stressful item ('death of a spouse': 100), is the same regardless of the individual's age, their dependence on the spouse, the length and happiness of the marriage, and so on. In addition, the model takes no account of how well the individual copes with any life event which occurs, or the support available from family or friends, to help them deal with it. The availability of such resources can provide a strong buffer against the psychological and physical effects of stressful life events (Cohen 1988).

Individual differences in stress response

What both the physiological model of Selye and the psychological model of Holmes and Rahe failed to explain were findings that only some individuals subject to apparently similar levels of stress become ill, or they develop different diseases (e.g. Cohen 1979). A number of more recent theories have attempted to explain these individual differences in response to stress. One, the diathesis-stress model (Levi 1974), proposed that while stressful events may form a trigger to the stress process, physiological predispositions towards a certain illness (such as a genetic weakness or chemical imbalance) and previously experienced environmental conditions are important determinants of the disease outcome. Evidence to support the diathesis-stress model can best be obtained by following individuals with an episodic stress-related disorder and observing whether this is exacerbated following or during periods of stress, and whether any other disease process occurs at these times. This type of study is rarely conducted, although what evidence there is does suggest some specificity of disease process (see Whitehead 1992). What is also evident is that not all individuals react to potentially stressful events in the same way.

A transactional model of stress

In one of the most influential models of stress, Lazarus and Folkman (1984) identified stress as a process in which environmental and cognitive events combine to determine behavioural, physiological, and psychological outcomes. The model is transactional, in that these processes are bi-directional. The environment may trigger a stress response, but the environment may, in turn, be modified by the individual to moderate, or exacerbate, its potential aversive effects.

Lazarus and Folkman stated that the first stage of the stress process is an environmental event, the meaning of which is considered by the individual. This process of appraisal has two elements. The first involves consideration of the event in terms of its potential psychological harm or challenge to the individual. If the event carries no threat potential, no further cognitive processing in terms of stress is conducted. If, however, the event carries the potential for harm, a second process of appraisal occurs in which the individual considers whether they have the resources to deal with the stressor. If the individual considers themselves capable of coping effectively with the threat the stress response is not activated. However, if they believe the demands of the situation to be greater than the resources they have available to cope with them, a stress process is initiated, involving the affective experience of stress (including feelings of anxiety or distress), sympathetically mediated arousal, and some form of stress-associated behaviour.

In order to reduce the aversive affective state associated with stress, Lazarus and Folkman suggest that we engage in a number of coping processes. Several specific coping responses have been identified, subsumed under two broad categories. Problem-focused coping involves the individual in active attempts to deal with, and change, the source of the stress. Emotion-focused coping involves the individual in attempts to reduce the negative emotional consequences of the stressor, but without addressing the initial cause of the stress. This may involve avoiding or not thinking about the cause of the stress, or behaviours such as drinking alcohol or smoking cigarettes. Most people do not exclusively engage in one set of coping strategies when dealing with a particular stressor, but may alternate between the two. Dependent on the effectiveness of these coping strategies, the original appraisal of the event may change and the stress process be exacerbated or moderated. The effectiveness of coping processes in moderating the impact of environmental stressors is a significantly greater predictor of health and illness than their frequency and apparent stressfulness (e.g. Cronkite and Moos 1984).

Stress as lack of control

While Lazarus and Folkman view stress as a process resulting from the interaction of environmental and person variables, their research has focused primarily on the person variables. Others have attempted to delineate aspects of the environment which are likely to result in stress. We have already noted that low socio-economic status is associated with high levels of environmental stressors. The workplace may also place considerable stress on the individual. Karasek and Theorell (1990), for example, identified two aspects of the work environment which appear to mediate stress and ill-health: the demands made on the individual by their job, and the degree of autonomy they are given to deal with these demands. These two factors work independently and together to predict work stress. Karasek argued that the most stressful combination of work circumstances are those which involve a high or excessive workload combined with a low level of job autonomy.

These circumstances may impact on all workers throughout the work hierarchy. Frankenhauser (1979), for example, found production line workers who could pace their own work had lower levels of stress hormones than those whose work rate was determined by machine. These differences can translate to health outcomes. Karasek et al. (1981) found that men who had jobs with low autonomy evidenced 40 per cent higher rates for CHD morbidity than those with high job control. In addition, men with highly demanding jobs evidenced 30 per cent higher morbidity than those in less demanding jobs. More recently, Johnson et al. (1996) followed a population of over 12,000 Swedish men for a period of 14 years. Workers in jobs defined as highly demanding and with low autonomy evidenced a risk for CHD double that for those in non-stressful jobs. If this high job stress was combined with a lack of support in the job, the risk increased to two and a half times that for those in low stress jobs.

Type A behaviour: a form of 'stressed' behaviour

Distortions in the appraisal and coping process play an important role in the development of a number of short-term psychological disorders such as depression and anxiety (Woolfolk and Lehrer 1993). They also underpin one, potentially life-long behavioural style, Type A behaviour, which is thought to place individuals at increased risk for CHD. In the next chapter, we examine some of the appraisal and coping processes thought to characterize this behavioural style. For now, we consider its association with CHD.

Type A behaviour, hostility, and CHD

Type A behaviour (TAB) is defined as an excess of free-floating hostility, competitiveness, and time urgency (Rosenman 1978). Its importance as a risk factor for CHD was first acknowledged after publication of the results of the Western Collaborative Group Study (WCGS: Rosenman et al. 1975).

This followed a population of 3,154 men, free of CHD, for a period initially of eight and a half years. Over this period, those assessed as Type A were found to carry twice the risk for CHD as those without these characteristics, so-called Type Bs, when other risk factors, such as smoking, were controlled for. Type A behaviour was more strongly linked to angina than MI, with the risk of disease in comparison to Type Bs being 2.5:1 and 2.1:1 respectively (Matthews and Haynes 1986). By the early 1980s, a number of other longitudinal studies, using differing measures of Type A behaviour, reported similar levels of association between Type A behaviour and CHD. This led a panel of eminent scientists (Review Panel 1981) to conclude that the risk for CHD conferred by TAB was of the same magnitude as that resulting from raised blood cholesterol, hypertension and smoking. More recently, the results of studies employing arguably less secure methodologies (e.g. Case et al. 1985; Shekelle et al. 1985) have apparently contradicted these conclusions (see Bennett 1994). However, they focused attention on one particular aspect of Type A behaviour, hostility, as being particularly implicated in the development of disease.

Re-analysis of the WCGS data (Chesney et al. 1988) showed the Type A components of anger and hostility to be more closely associated with disease than overall ratings of Type A behaviour. This close association was reinforced by the findings of the MRFIT study (Dembroski et al. 1989) where hostility, but not Type A behaviour, predicted the incidence of MI. Accordingly, the present consensus is that while Type A behaviour may predict CHD in some individuals, the relationship between hostility and anger with the development of CHD is more substantial.

Hostility and Type A behaviour are thought to exert their influence on health through frequent or excessive increases in blood pressure within the coronary arteries consequent to high levels of sympathetic activation. These occur during episodes of anger or Type A behaviour and may damage the artery walls, resulting in increased deposition of atheroma. High levels of catecholamines driving the sympathetic activation also increase platelet stickiness and increase risk for the production of blood clots (Markovitz and Matthews 1991). Krantz and Durel (1983) have argued that this hyper-reactivity may be constitutional in nature, and that physiological reactivity drives behavioural reactivity. Others (e.g. Price 1988) have argued that these behaviours and affective states, and their associated high arousal are the consequence of social learning (see chapter 2, this volume). The latter provides some optimism for change. If these are learned behaviours, they can be unlearned and replaced with new behaviours. However, in view of their prevalence throughout the population (about half of those assessed are rated Type A), changing all those who exhibit these behaviours may be unwarranted. Accordingly, it may only be worth intervening to change these behaviours in individuals who carry other risks for CHD (Bennett et al. 1991c), or who have already evidenced heart disease (Friedman et al. 1986).

Changing behaviour: two cautionary tales

Health promotion has implicitly assumed that changing factors known to contribute to risk for disease will in some way modify that risk and, in time, reduce the incidence of disease. This seems a reasonable assumption. However, it has not always been substantiated in studies examining the impact of changes in serum cholesterol and blood pressure on morbidity and mortality.

An editorial in the *British Medical Journal* (Marmot 1994) was subtitled, somewhat enigmatically, 'Lowering population cholesterol concentrations probably isn't harmful'. In this article, Marmot noted that a 0.6 mmol/litre reduction of cholesterol throughout the population should theoretically be associated with a 27 per cent reduction in mortality from CHD. However, evidence from a number of treatment trials suggests that while death rates from coronary heart disease may be reduced following interventions to reduce serum cholesterol levels, all cause mortality rates to appear unchanged. The reasons for this remain unclear. Reduced levels of cholesterol through dietary and drug manipulation have been associated with an increased incidence of cancer (Muldoon *et al.* 1991), although this finding is not universal (Burr *et al.* 1989). In addition, modest differences in non-illness-related mortality, including suicide, accidents and violence (Muldoon *et al.* 1991) have also followed reductions in blood cholesterol levels. These data suggest that intervening to reduce cholesterol levels at a population level may not bring about the universal reductions in morbidity initially expected, and some (Davey Smith and Pekkanen 1992) have called for a moratorium to be called on all such initiatives.

However, such a negative approach may be premature, as these risks appear to be differentially distributed throughout the population. In a meta-analysis of data from 36 large-scale clinical trials, Davey Smith *et al.* (1993) found that the value of treatment was linked to initial levels of cholesterol: among people with high serum cholesterol levels intervention was beneficial; in those with moderately raised cholesterol levels no benefit was found; in those with low levels intervention was actually deleterious, with higher overall mortality rates in the intervention than control groups. However, this later finding was only found for interventions using drug treatments. For those trials using dietary methods, those in the low risk group did not run any increase in risk. In addition, levels of cholesterol reduction resulting from dietary change matched those of drug treatment. Accordingly, dietary change as a means of changing population levels of serum cholesterol appears to be highly appropriate and safe.

A similar picture may be emerging for the treatment of mild hypertension. While risk for coronary heart disease and stroke is proportionate to levels of blood pressure, the highest morbidity to these diseases is found among people with only mildly or moderately raised blood pressure, because there are so many of them. In the MRFIT study (Stamler 1990), for example, those with high–normal pressures accounted for about a quarter of the excess cardiovascular deaths related to above optimal blood pressure. Even relatively small reductions in blood pressures of 5 mmHg should lower coronary death rates by 9 per cent, stroke by 14 per cent and all deaths by 7 per cent (Collins *et al.* 1990). While drug treatment of this population has reduced pressures, these reductions have not yielded the expected benefits of disease reduction (Collins *et al.* 1990), perhaps as a consequence of the negative effects of anti-hypertensive drugs on blood lipids and glucose metabolism.

An alternative approach which should yield similar reductions in blood pressure may be the control of blood pressure through reductions in salt and potassium intake, weight, and alcohol consumption. Such a change may result from both individual behavioural change and changes in the constituents of processed food; 75 per cent of the sodium intake in countries such as the USA and UK is from processed food (NRC 1989) and change here could result in significant reductions in consumption.

Behaviour change programmes have also proven effective. Stamler *et al.* (1989), for example, allocated overweight hypertension-prone individuals to either a monitoring condition or one in which they were asked to eat a low fat diet, reduce their alcohol intake to two drinks per day, and increase their exercise to three periods of 30 minutes per week. Although only a minority of participants achieved all the dietary and behavioural goals set, during the five years of the trial the incidence of hypertension was more than twice as high in a control group as in the intervention group (19.2 versus 8.8 per cent). Similar findings have been replicated in non-medicated populations (e.g. HPT Research Group 1990) and in stable medicated hypertensives (Stamler *et al.* 1986).

These data provide encouraging evidence of the value of health promotion. Although changes in risk factors may be achieved through some form of pharmaceutical intervention, any changes achieved are likely to be costly and may not translate to reduced risk for disease. Conversely, the effects of health promotion are relatively cheap, carry no adverse side-effects, and seem to be more effective in some populations than medical intervention.

Summary and conclusions

There is clear evidence that health status is not simply mediated by biological factors, but is affected by social, economic, psychological and societal processes. Individually mediated behaviours such as diet, exercise and smoking may directly affect health. Social class and gender also impact directly on health. However, a significant variance in health status is attributable to an interaction between behavioural and societal processes. Low socio-economic status is associated with environmental stress. It may also be associated with a lack of resources through which to mitigate the effect of such stressors or through which to engage in health promoting behaviours, poor access to appropriate health care resources, and so on. Gender specific roles may influence uptake of exercise and job autonomy. In addition, family processes may influence a wide range of health-related behaviours (see Murphy and Bennett 1994).

Health and health-related behaviours occur within a complex system of interacting influences. Accordingly, effective health promotion should address the system, and not just isolated individuals within it. This will require multi-level interventions, focused on individuals, societal processes (and those such as politicians, who control such processes), environmental and cultural processes.

Suggested reading

Amler, R.W. and Dull, H.B. (1987) *Closing the Gap: The Burden of Unnecessary Illness*. New York: Oxford University Press.

Carroll, D., Davey Smith, G. and Bennett, P. (1996) Social class and health: the widening gap. *Journal of Health Psychology*, 1: 23–39.

Lazarus, R.S. and Folkman, S. (1984) *Stress, Appraisal, and Coping*. New York: Springer Publications.

Reddy, D.M., Fleming, R. and Adesso, V.J. (1992) Gender and health. In S. Maes, H. Leventhal and M. Johnston (eds) *International Review of Health Psychology, Volume 1*. Chichester: Wiley.

Smith, A. and Jacobson, B. (eds) (1988) *The Nation's Health. A Strategy for the 1990s*. London: King's Fund Centre.

Cognitive mediators of health-related behaviours

Present psychological theory is premised on the assumption that cognitive processes mediate behaviour. As yet, no superordinate theory of decision-making, able to identify and integrate all of these processes, has emerged. Instead, a number of theories are being developed, each focusing on different aspects of this process. Those relevant to health promotion include both general theories of behavioural decision-making and those which focus specifically on health-related behaviours. In this chapter we describe and evaluate some of the more influential models, examining their historical antecedents and their explanatory power. In doing so, we first introduce two early models of the acquisition and maintenance of behaviour which assumed, in contrast to our present theories, that behaviour was governed solely by environmental factors, not by internal, cognitive, processes. We then explore more cognitively based theories.

Conditioning theory

Classical conditioning

In the early 1900s Ivan Pavlov, a Russian physiologist, developed what many consider to be the first 'scientific' explanation of behaviour. While studying the physiology of digestion, he noticed that his laboratory dogs began to salivate as he entered the laboratory carrying their empty food dishes. He surmised that the dogs had in some way learned an association between seeing the dish and being fed, and were responding to the dish as if it contained food. He was later able to demonstrate this phenomenon as reliable and applicable to a wide variety of responses and stimuli (Pavlov 1927). In a typical experiment, he would present an animal with a stimulus which elicited a natural physiological response: salivation to the presentation of food, fear or avoidant behaviour in the case of a painful stimulus, and so on. At the same time another event, such as a ringing bell or flashing light would occur. Over repeated presentations, this event took on the same properties as the first stimulus, eliciting a response almost identical to the initial one – in the above cases, a salivation or fear response. Based on these findings, he developed a law of classical conditioning which stated that an unconditioned stimulus (e.g. food) if frequently associated with a conditioned stimulus (e.g. a bell), will come to elicit a conditioned response, which closely resembles the unconditioned one. If this association no longer occurs, the conditioned response will continue for some time, but become less strong and eventually cease, a process known as extinction.

Pavlov considered conditioning took place at a visceral level, and was not mediated by cognitive processes. He also stated that this type of learning is the same in all species, and is one of the building blocks for more complex learning. Conditioning processes, for example, contribute to the development of many phobias and obsessional behaviours. Both can be conditioned fear responses (see Bandura 1969). Fear of the dentist may follow a particularly painful procedure; fear of cars may follow involvement in an accident. In each case, the fear felt at the time of the original event is evoked subsequently in the presence of a similar stimulus, frequently leading to its avoidance.

Classical conditioning explains how behaviours already in an animal's repertoire can be linked to previously unrelated stimuli. It cannot explain how we learn new behaviours. For this, a different class of learning experiences is required: that of operant conditioning (Skinner 1953).

Operant conditioning

Operant theory states that behaviour that is rewarded, or reinforced, will continue or increase in frequency. Behaviour that is punished will reduce in frequency or cease. These definitions are empirically derived: that which increases behaviour is, by definition, a reinforcer; that which decreases behaviour, a punisher. A third process, known as negative reinforcement, occurs when an individual avoids an aversive stimulus, and is thus 'rewarded', through engaging in some form of behaviour.

Reinforcement processes are important mediators of the uptake and maintenance of many health-related behaviours. New smokers, for example, frequently gain social reinforcement from their peers as a consequence of their smoking. Later in their smoking career, they are rewarded for smoking cigarettes through the changes in mood and attention within seconds of inhalation (Ashton and Stepney 1982). Conversely, when many individuals quit smoking they experience withdrawal effects which are alleviated by smoking a further cigarette: a process of negative reinforcement. In fact, behaviour frequently results in a variety of potentially reinforcing or punishing outcomes. Young smokers, for example, may experience both peer reinforcement for their smoking and disapproval or punishment from their parents. In such cases, Skinner argued that the closer the reward or punishment to the behaviour, the more this contingency controls it.

Operant theory provides a powerful explanation of much of our behaviour, but it has a number of limitations. These stem from the radical nature of Skinner's theory, which stated that behaviour is a consequence of behaviour–reward interactions, and is not mediated by cognitive processes. Skinner considered such processes to be 'epiphenomena', in that they are clearly experienced, but do not mediate behaviour. Such radicalism led to a number of critiques. From a philosophical perspective, many objected to the lack of free will implied by Skinner's writings. From a phenomenological perspective, it seemed difficult to accept that our thoughts did not, at some times at least, guide behaviour. From a theoretical perspective, Skinner's theory had a number of difficulties in explaining the development of long-term goals and plans, the acquisition of language, and how we learn through observation of others. What became clear was that while much of our behaviour could be attributed to our experience of rewards and punishments, this relationship was mediated by symbolic, or cognitive, processes.

Social learning theory

While not rejecting some of the principles of behaviourism, more recent theories have extended learning principles to include cognitive processes. The most influential of these has been social learning theory, or social cognitive theory as it later became known (Bandura 1977, 1986).

Social cognitive theory states that behaviour is the outcome of an interaction between cognitive processes and environmental events. As in operant conditioning theory, the individual is still motivated to gain the maximum reinforcement and minimum punishment from their environment. However, behaviours are considered not just to be governed by immediate behaviour–consequence contingencies. Rather, the individual is able to defer gratification and actively plan and work towards short and long-term behavioural goals based upon choices between differentially valued reinforcers, behavioural outcomes learned from observation of others, and a moral framework. Three elements of social cognitive theory are particularly relevant to health promotion, and will be examined here in some detail: the role of expectancies in determining behaviour, the process of vicarious learning, and the motivating influence of good health as a behavioural outcome.

The role of expectancies

Behaviour is goal oriented. According to Bandura, the individual is motivated to engage in behaviours whose outcome is valued and which they feel capable of performing effectively. Behavioural choice is premised on two sets of expectancies. The first, action–outcome expectancies, reflect the degree to which individuals believe that an action will lead to a particular outcome: 'smoking causes cancer', 'stopping smoking reduces the risk of cancer', and so on. This outcome is then considered in terms of its value to the individual. The second set of expectancies, self-efficacy expectations, reflect the extent to which individuals believe themselves capable of the behaviour being considered: 'I can give up smoking', 'I'm not sure whether I can give up smoking at present', and so on. According to this decision-making process, the smoker will only attempt to quit smoking if they believe that smoking cessation will reduce their risk for disease, place a high value on this behavioural outcome, and believe they are capable of doing so.

Efficacy beliefs operate at different levels. Generalized efficacy beliefs ('I can cope with most things life throws at me') may moderate a variety of behaviours, and are relevant when the individual is faced with a unique behavioural decision. However, behaviour-specific efficacy beliefs are frequently more powerful determinants of behaviour. Marlatt et al. (1994), for example, identified a number of efficacy judgements relevant to different stages of drug and alcohol misuse. The first, resistance self-efficacy beliefs, reflect the confidence the individual has in their ability to avoid substance abuse prior to its first use. Harm-reduction self-efficacy beliefs involve judgements of ability to reduce the risks of drug use once initiated. Action self-efficacy beliefs refer to the individual's confidence in attaining abstinence or controlled consumption. Coping self-efficacy beliefs relate to their being able to avoid relapse. Finally, recovery self-efficacy beliefs reflect the individual's perceived ability to recover from any relapse.

Outcome and efficacy beliefs have been shown to be important moderators of a number of health-related behaviours including resisting peer pressure to smoke or use drugs (Stacy et al. 1992), weight loss (Bagozzi and Warshaw 1990), engaging in safer sex practices (McKusick et al. 1990; O'Leary et al. 1992), and breast self-examination (Rippetoe and Rogers 1987). In the context of drug use, Kok et al. (1992) reported a study in which they analysed the use of condoms and clean needles by drug addicts in Amsterdam. Perceived self-efficacy correlated with intentions to use clean needles, reported clean needle use, intentions to use condoms and reported condom use. Dzewaltowski et al. (1990) similarly found adherence to a prescribed exercise regime to be correlated with perceived self-efficacy, outcome expectancies and dissatisfaction with previous levels of fitness. Individuals who were confident that they could adhere to the strenuous exercise programme and who were dissatisfied with their present level of physical activity exercised the most. Finally, from work on smoking cessation, efficacy beliefs concerning the ability to resist smoking having quit have been shown to predict the numbers of cigarettes smoked, the amount of tobacco per cigarette and nicotine levels (Godding and Glasgow 1985). Here, the stronger participants' beliefs in their ability to quit, the less they smoked.

Such is the influence of outcome and efficacy beliefs on behaviour, that Schwarzer (1994) has suggested that these form the major determinants of many health-related behaviours (see 'the health action process', below). If so, health promotion initiatives may benefit from changing efficacy beliefs. One method of doing so is through teaching strategies or skills relevant to any desired behavioural change. Vicarious learning and modelling provide one route through which this can be achieved.

Vicarious learning and modelling

Many of the behaviours we engage in are a consequence of the behavioural models we have been exposed to over the life course. From observing such models, we vicariously learn behavioural outcomes and establish efficacy expectancies without necessarily having direct experience of these ourselves. These processes provide a more cogent explanation of the uptake and main-tenance of many health-related behaviours than operant theory from which it was derived. For example, we noted earlier in this chapter that peer rein-forcement provides a powerful reward to the uptake of smoking. However, the initial experience of smoking is highly aversive. Operant theory states that this powerful punishment, directly associated with the act of smoking, should lead to an immediate cessation of such behaviour. Yet this is clearly not the case for many young people. The process of vicarious learning affords an explanation. This suggests that at the same time the individual experiences aversive consequences to smoking, they also observe in others that smok-ing can be a pleasurable and rewarding behaviour, so they persevere in the expectation of future enjoyment. In the language of social learning theory, the young smoker learns from the observation of others, and forms behavi-oural plans on the basis of valued future action–outcome expectations.

Families and peers provide strong modelling influences on young persons; those who smoke, for example, are more likely to have family and friends who do so (Ashton and Stepney 1982). The media also provides an enormous number of models of behaviour, not all of them positive. Consider, for example, the high levels of risky sex practices portrayed on television and in films. In general, people are more likely to perform the behaviour they observe if the model is similar to themselves; that is, of the same sex, age, or race (see Chapter 6, this volume). In addition, high status persons, either from within the social sphere of the individual, or from wider spheres such as sports or the media exert a stronger influence on behaviour than low status individuals (Winett et al. 1989). The process of modelling provides a strong entry point for health promotion programmes. High status indi-viduals modelling health promoting behaviour can encourage others to copy their behaviour. Modelling may also be used to teach skills necessary to achieve behavioural change, or increase efficacy expectations through seeing others attempting and succeeding in change.

Good health as a valued outcome?

Good health forms an action–outcome expectancy and, if valued, a possible reward for engaging in health-maintaining or promoting behaviour. It is a probabilistic outcome; engaging in health-maintaining behaviour reduces, but does not eliminate, the risk of disease. It is also a long-term outcome; very few, if any, health-related behaviours have an immediate and notice-able effect on health. In addition, the motivation to work towards the long-term goal of good health frequently competes with a plethora of short-term rewards for behaving in health-damaging ways. Not surprisingly, these short-term rewards are frequently more powerful influences on behaviour than the promise of long-term good health. Indeed, a significant percentage of individuals engage in harmful behaviour in order to 'look good'. Findings from a survey cited in Klesges *et al.* (1989), for example, indicated that about a third of young adult smokers use their smoking as a means of controlling their weight. A smaller percentage of smokers (10 per cent men, 5 per cent women) actually start smoking in order to do so. Weight gain is also a significant factor in relapse, especially among females, and may act as a significant barrier to future cessation attempts (Klesges *et al.* 1989).

Even where good health is highly valued, lapses in behaviour can be justi-fied through a variety of cognitive processes, including denial ('My old gran lived to 103, and smoked 20 Woodbines every day of her life') or some form of bargaining ('I'll eat that ice cream now, but I'll eat more healthily tomorrow'). Short-term 'health' outcomes may be much more powerful determinants of behaviour. Looking fit and being able to get into attractive clothes, for example, may be more important determinants of success in dieting than any long-term health gains (Norman and Bennett 1996).

Health locus of control

Locus of control beliefs reflect the extent to which an individual believes that their actions will result in desired outcomes. In this, it is a similar construct to self-efficacy. Rotter (1966) divided individuals into 'internals' and 'externals'. According to this typology, internals believe that events are a consequence of their actions, and consequently under personal control. Externals, in contrast, believe that events are unrelated to their actions and determined by factors beyond their personal control.

In a more complex model specific to health, Wallston *et al.* (1978) identi-fied three statistically independent dimensions of perceived control: internal, chance, and powerful others. Their model suggests that those who score highly on the internal dimension regard their health as largely within their own control and are likely to engage in health-maintaining behaviours. Conversely, those who score highly on the chance dimension view their health as relatively independent of their behaviour and, accordingly, are more likely to engage in health-damaging behaviours than those with lower scores. The implications of a strong belief in powerful others (typically doctors) influencing health are more difficult to predict. High ratings may indicate a receptivity to health messages endorsed by medical authorities. Conversely, they may suggest a strong belief in the ability of the medical system to cure any relevant illness and a consequent disregard for health promotion messages.

In accord with social learning theory, from which it was developed, Wallston (e.g. Wallston and Smith 1994) stated that individuals are motivated to engage in behaviours which lead to valued outcomes. Health locus of control beliefs will only influence the health-related behaviours of those who place a high value on their health. People are unlikely to engage in health protective behaviours, whatever their locus of control beliefs, if they do not value their health. Accordingly, those most likely to engage in health enhancing behaviours are people who place a high value on their health and who score highly on measures of internal health locus of control.

Health locus of control theory has been one of the most influential in health psychology, and has generated a large body of research. However, the association between locus of control scales and health-related behaviours has been surprisingly modest. In a series of studies based on a representative British population sample of over 13,000 people (e.g. Bennett *et al.* 1995; 1997), we found locus of control and value for health dimensions to predict, at most, only 5 per cent of the variance in measures of exercise, smoking, diet, alcohol consumption and a composite lifestyle measure, even among respondents placing a high value on their health.

These data are in accord with much of the research conducted on smaller samples. Here, research outcomes have been mixed, with both positive (e.g. Weiss and Larsen 1990) and negative (e.g. Steptoe *et al.* 1994) findings. Slenker *et al.* (1985), for example, found joggers to have higher internal health locus of control scores than non-joggers. Conversely, Calnan (1989) found no relationship between exercise and internal health locus of control scores in a large British population sample. Kelly *et al.* (1990) found gay men who reported having unprotected anal intercourse were less likely to have internal AIDS-related locus of control beliefs and more likely to believe that the likelihood of HIV infection was attributable to chance factors. In contrast, St Lawrence (1993) found no relationship between internal beliefs and the use of condoms in a sample of African-American adolescents. Similarly mixed findings in other health domains have led Wallston to draw a number of pessimistic conclusions about the ability of the health locus of control construct alone to predict preventive health behaviour (Wallston and Wallston 1984).

Attitude and attitude change theory

Attitudes are likes and dislikes, frequently expressed as opinion statements. They have two components: a belief about an object, behaviour

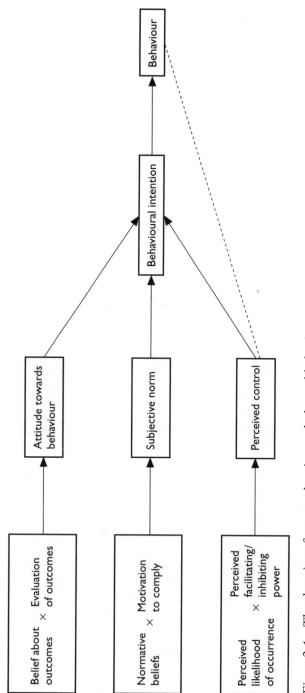

Figure 2.1 The theories of reasoned action and planned behaviour

or behavioural outcome ('I believe that eating fruit will help maintain health'; 'Some apples are coloured red'), and an evaluative component. This involves an appraisal of the belief in terms of its value to the individual ('I value keeping healthy'; 'I like the taste of red apples'). An individual may hold a number of, perhaps conflicting, attitudes towards any one behaviour or issue, with the sum of these forming their overall attitude.

Early attitudinal research assumed a strong relationship between attitudes and behaviour, and many early health promotion programmes were premised on the belief that changing attitudes would lead to behavioural change. Implicit in these approaches were theories such as cognitive dissonance theory (Festinger 1957). This stated that attitude and behavioural change can be achieved by providing information counter to the attitudes presently held by an individual. The state of mental discomfort so created, known as cognitive dissonance, acted as a motivator either to reject the new information or to adopt attitudes and behaviours more consonant with the new information. However, there is substantial evidence that attitudes are only, at best, moderately related to behaviour. An early, but classic, study conducted by LaPiere (1934) illustrates the point. LaPiere travelled through the USA with a Chinese couple, booking into over 200 motels and restaurants. At the time there was strong anti-Asian prejudice in the USA and no legislation to prevent discrimination in public accommodation. Nevertheless, only one establishment refused to allow them a room. LaPiere then wrote to each establishment asking them whether they would accept a Chinese couple as guests. Of the 128 which replied, 92 per cent said no – a statement clearly at odds with their behaviour.

Despite the modest relationship between attitudes and behaviour, attitudes still form an important subject for psychological research. Some attitudinal theorists (e.g. Petty and Cacioppo 1986, see Chapter 6, pages 99–101) have attempted to further delineate the mechanisms of attitudinal change and how this may be manipulated. Others have combined attitudes with other variables in order to develop more predictive models. Elaborations of attitudinal theory have involved adding components including intentions to behave, social influences (Fishbein and Ajzen 1975), and the perceived availability of the desired behaviour (Ajzen 1985). These theories are now examined in more detail.

Theories of reasoned action and planned behaviour

The theory of reasoned action (Ajzen and Fishbein 1980, see Figure 2.1) states that the primary determinant of behaviour is an intention to engage in that behaviour. Behavioural intentions are derived from two parallel cognitive processes. The first involves consideration of the individual's own attitudes towards the behaviour. The second involves consideration of the relevant social norms. Attitudes comprise beliefs about the behaviour under consideration, and valences attached to those beliefs. Social norms also comprise two elements: an appraisal of the likelihood that salient others would wish the individual to engage (or not) in the behaviour under consideration, and their motivation to comply with these expectations. 'Salient others' typically includes friends or other people whose opinions are important to the individual.

An assumption of the theory of reasoned action is that the individual has the resources, skills, or opportunities to engage in their desired action. This is frequently not the case, and to address this weakness Ajzen (1985) added a further dimension: that of control over the intended behaviour. This reflects the perceived ability of the individual to engage in the desired behaviour. Facilitating or inhibiting factors include both internal (skills, information, and so on) and external control factors (including opportunities and dependence on others). Perceived control combines with attitudes and perceived norms to form an intention to engage in a particular behaviour. This larger model is termed the theory of planned behaviour (Ajzen 1985).

The theories of reasoned action and planned behaviour are general models of behavioural decision-making, and have been applied to behaviours as varied as lying, cheating and shoplifting as well as the less morally dubious behaviours of dealing in stocks and shares. They have also been used to predict a number of health-related behaviours, including smoking initiation (Sutton 1989), condom use (Terry et al. 1993), oral contraceptive use (Doll and Orth 1993), and participation in exercise (Norman and Smith 1995). Reviews of the theory of reasoned action literature (Sheppard et al. 1988; van den Putte 1993) suggest the model has substantial predictive utility, with multiple correlations for attitudes and perceived social norms with intentions averaging between 0.66 and 0.68. Adding perceived control to the model increases its predictive utility only slightly. In a review of 16 studies, Ajzen (1991) reported the average multiple correlation between intentions and all three dimensions to be 0.71. The strength of association between intentions and behaviour is somewhat lower, with mean correlations averaging between 0.45 (Randall and Wolff 1994) and 0.62 (van den Putte 1993). The strength of this relationship may vary considerably according to behaviour, with correlations between intentions and measures of behaviour varying between 0.01 to 0.94 (Sheppard et al. 1988; Conner et al. 1994). About 10 per cent of studies report correlations below 0.2 (Sheppard et al. 1988).

Some of the more disappointing results may reflect experimental inadequacies (see Norman and Conner 1996). Others may reflect a failure of the model to address factors, such as contextual variables, which may also impact on decision-making. An interesting example of how intentions may not translate into action is reported by Abraham et al. (1995) in the context of condom use by adolescents and young adults. Among these groups, the correlation between intentions to use condoms during intercourse and their actual use was significant for men but not for women, reflecting findings of qualitative studies (e.g. Holland et al. 1990) that young women are frequently disempowered in sexual negotiation, so that their behavioural intentions are not translated into action.

Health belief model

The health belief model (Becker 1974; see Figure 2.2) focuses on two related appraisal processes: the threat of illness, and the behavioural response to that threat. Threat appraisal involves consideration of both the individual's perceived susceptibility to an illness and its anticipated severity. Behavioural evaluation involves consideration of the costs and benefits of engaging in behaviours likely to reduce the threat of disease. In addition, the model suggests that health-related decisions are triggered by environmental cues. Later versions of the model (Becker 1974) added a fourth dimension, the individual's motivation or 'readiness to be concerned about health matters', although this has rarely been addressed by researchers (Conner and Norman 1996). Although each factor is considered of importance in any decision-making process, no clear operationalization of how the constructs combine to result in a final decision has been developed (see Ronis and Harel 1989; Lewis 1994). Accordingly, the model is operationalized as six variables, each independently contributing to the decision-making process.

According to the health belief model, the decision whether or not to use a condom with a new partner, for example, would involve consideration of a number of issues. Threat perception would involve consideration of how likely the individual is to encounter an HIV-positive lover, the risk of HIV transmission through unprotected sex, and the severity of any subsequent illness. Behavioural evaluation involves consideration of the likelihood of safer sexual practices reducing risk of viral transmission, and the costs of doing so. The former may reflect concerns about the effectiveness of condoms. The latter may include the potential embarrassment of purchasing condoms or negotiating their use, lessening the pleasure of sex, and so on. Finally, the salience of condom use may differ according to the individual's experiences of HIV infection, AIDS, or health promotion programmes concerning safer sex.

Significant associations between dimensions of the health belief model and behaviours as varied as engaging in exercise programmes (Langie 1977), child vaccination (Bennett and Smith 1992), compliance with recommended medical regimes (Bradley and Kegeles 1987) and attending preventive screening clinics (Orbell et al. 1995) have been reported. In a review of 46 studies, Janz and Becker (1984) reported that measures of susceptibility were significantly associated with health behaviours in 82 per cent of studies, measures of perceived severity in 65 per cent, benefits in 81 per cent, and costs in 100 per cent. However, while consistent associations between health belief model dimensions and behaviour have been found, the magnitude of these relationships is generally low.

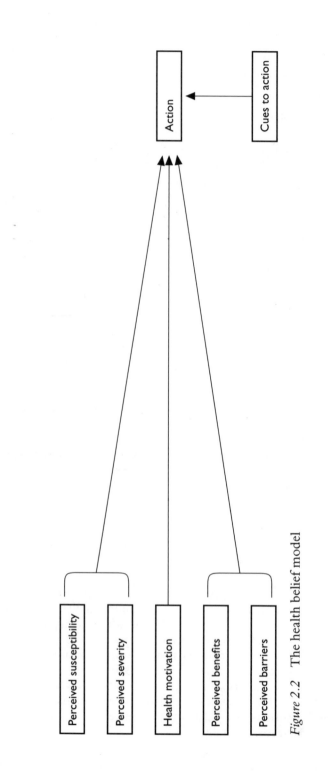

Figure 2.2 The health belief model

Using meta-analytical techniques to combine data from a number of studies, Harrison *et al.* (1992) found average correlations between health belief model dimensions and behaviour to be modest at best: 0.15 for susceptibility, 0.08 for severity, 0.13 for benefits, and −0.21 for barriers. Individual components of the health belief model accounted for an average of between 0.5 and 4 per cent of the variance in behaviour across studies. However, Harrison *et al.* (1992) failed to combine the factors to measure their combined predictive power, as the model suggests. In addition, they reported highly variable results from different studies, suggesting that for some behaviours the predictive utility of the health belief model may be much stronger than their overall results would suggest.

The predictive utility of cues to action has been less evaluated. Physicians' advice has been found to influence smoking cessation (Stacy and Lloyd 1990) and postcard prompts to attend screening increase attendance (Norman and Conner 1993). However, Wolcott *et al.* (1990) found that knowing someone with HIV infection or AIDS was not predictive of behavioural change among gay men. Overall, evidence that cues to action have a consistent impact on motivation and behavioural choice is lacking, although this may be a result of a failure to measure the construct effectively (Sheeran and Abraham 1996).

Stage theories

The models described so far implicitly assume that each cognitive process involved in decision-making occurs in roughly the same time frame and in parallel. However, more recent work has suggested that there may be qualitatively different stages in such processing, with the content of cognitions varying with time.

One of the first 'stages of change' models was proposed by Prochaska and DiClemente (1984). Their transtheoretical model identified five stages through which people pass when moving towards behavioural change: pre-contemplation, contemplation, preparation, action, and maintenance or relapse. In the pre-contemplation stage, change is not being considered. In the contemplation stage, the individual is considering change at some remote level but is not yet committed to change, and has not thought through how this may be achieved. As the individual moves to the preparation stage, they begin actively considering and planning change. As its name implies, the action stage is when behavioural change actually occurs. However, only after about two months is any behavioural change considered significantly established to be considered in the maintenance stage. Individuals who reach the action stage may fail to maintain any changes made, and relapse back to any one of the previous stages. The model is cyclic and bi-directional; individuals involved in behavioural change may start at any point in the process, and progress or move back to an earlier stage at any time. The processes which

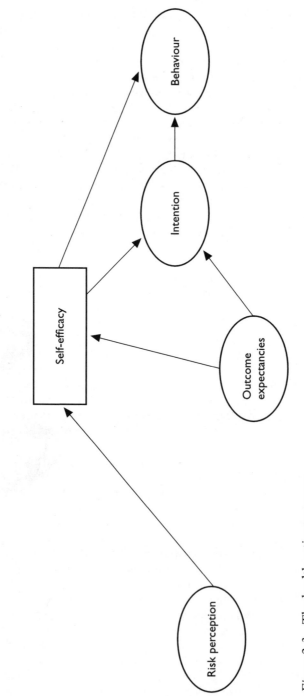

Figure 2.3   The health action process

facilitate these transitions are less considered by the model. However, they may be highly idiosyncratic: an illness, a friend changing their behaviour, and so on.

A similar process of change has been described by Heckhausen (1991), who identified four stages of change: pre-decisional, post-decisional, actional and evaluative. In addition, Heckhausen suggested that the content of cognitions differed between each stage. In the pre-decisional phase, cognitions concerning the desirability and feasibility of a new behaviour predominate and may result in an intention to change. The decisional phase begins with consideration of plans for behavioural change and ends with the successful initiation of the new behaviour. In the final, evaluative phase, the individual is thought to compare achieved outcomes with initial goals in order to regulate and maintain behaviour.

The health action process

A further theoretical model combines many of the processes previously described, placing them in the context of a stage theory. The health action process (Schwarzer 1992; see Figure 2.3) states that the adoption of health-related behaviours involves two stages: a motivational and volitional stage. The latter is further subdivided into planning, action, and maintenance phases.

The motivational stage is triggered by the perception of a threat to health. However, unlike some expectancy value models (e.g. Becker 1974), Schwarzer argues that only a minimum level of threat or concern is required to initiate consideration of change. More important are action–outcome expectancies and self-efficacy judgements; that is, consideration of how risk may be reduced and whether the required actions are within the capabilities of the individual. Consideration of action–outcome expectancies temporally precedes self-efficacy judgements; people usually make assumptions about the possible consequences of a behaviour before considering engaging in that behaviour. The outcome of these deliberations may be an intention to adopt a precaution measure or to change risk behaviours in favour of other behaviours.

Once an intention is determined, the individual moves to the action phase. This involves a move to detailed consideration of how an intentional goal may be achieved. A global intention (for example, to lose weight) is specified in a set of subordinate intentions and action plans that contain proximal goals and algorithms for action sequences (lose 2lb per week, eat differing foods, etc.). This process is relatively unaffected by outcome expectancies, and more strongly by self-efficacy expectations, as the number and quality of action plans are strongly dependent on one's perceived competence and experience. However, the more plans and contingencies are considered, the more likely is behavioural change.

Once an action has been initiated, it has to be controlled by cognitions in order to be maintained. Again, Schwarzer argues that self-efficacy judgements determine the amount of effort and perseverance invested in the new behaviour. Finally, the context in which change is attempted will influence its outcome. Actions are not just the result of cognitions, but are controlled by the perceived and actual environment. Changes which are supported by the social and structural environment are more likely to be maintained than those which are not.

The importance of outcome and efficacy judgements in determining behavioural change has been established earlier in the chapter. The newer elements of Schwarzer's theory have not yet received substantial scientific enquiry and their predictive utility is yet to be determined. However, in common with a number of other theories (Bagozzi and Warshaw 1990; Gollwitzer 1993), the model provides the potential to understand more fully the modest association between intentions and behaviour.

Risk perception and dispositional optimism

The perception of personal vulnerability to disease is an important initiator of preventive behaviours. Accordingly, many health promotion programmes have attempted to raise awareness of the risks to health associated with certain behaviours. When faced with such information, the individual is faced with the task of deciding the magnitude and relevance of that risk to them. Most people do not have, or indeed want, access to unbiased or full information through which to arrive at a considered judgement. Instead they resort to a series of heuristics, or 'rules of thumb' (Kahneman et al. 1982). Such a process frequently involves the simplification of new risk information and comparison with those which are more familiar.

Heuristics involve consistent biases (Tversky and Kahneman 1982). Risk outcomes that are encountered frequently or carry a high threat value are likely to be attended to (Weinstein 1984). Conversely, where the probability of an event is low, any degree of risk may be dismissed altogether and considered as a risk hardly worth worrying about (Douglas 1986). Even where risk appraisal is based on appropriate information, perceived risks can still be moderated by so-called irrational factors. Davidson et al. found that while a majority of respondents in a large scale community survey understood that heart disease was to some extent preventable or postponable, 'the idea that it could happen to anyone (at any time) was omnipresent' (1991: 14). Such a belief mitigated much of the preventive message that they had understood.

Over-optimistic biases in evaluating personal health risk are common. Biases based on inappropriate temporal (Taylor 1989) and social (Weinstein 1980) comparisons are particularly prevalent. Temporal comparison biases typically minimize the probability of an adverse health event in the future.

Social comparison biases involve differences in perceived risk, favouring oneself in comparison to others ('Smoking may damage other people's health, but not mine'). These biases have been found for perceived risk of HIV infection, high cholesterol, MI, lung cancer, and liver cirrhosis (Van der Velde *et al.* 1992; Schwarzer 1994). Such over-optimism may deter individuals from engaging in appropriate health protective behaviours, and may need to be addressed in any health promotion initiative.

Cognitive models of health-related decision-making: a critique

The theories outlined provide a parsimonious description of at least some of the processes involved in health-related decision-making. Together, they have provided a theoretical foundation for a number of innovative and important health promotion initiatives targeted at both individuals and communities (e.g. Puska *et al.* 1985; Maccoby 1988). Nevertheless, they each have some weaknesses, and their implications for health promotion have been questioned. Accordingly, we finish this chapter with a brief critical appraisal of some of the principles underlying the models and their application in health promotion. In doing so, we address three issues: the routine nature of much of our behaviour; alternative 'rationalities' to maintaining health; and cultural and social influences on health behaviour. Some of these are returned to again in Chapter 8.

Behavioural 'thoughtlessness' and post hoc rationalizations

The central assumption of all expectancy-value theories is that behaviour is the outcome of a formal decision-making process. This need not take place each time an individual engages in a health-related behaviour: rather, the outcome of the decision-making process is held in memory and enacted upon as appropriate. Indeed, much of our behaviour appears to be routine and relatively 'thoughtless' (Hunt and Martin 1988).

Perhaps the most startling evidence of this comes from a study of working-class households reported by Cullen (1979). Their respondents considered 90 per cent of their waking day to involve no real choices but, rather, an adaptation to a relatively stable long-term environment. Further relevant evidence was reported by Bremble *et al.* (1991), who interviewed a group of middle-aged people about their dietary habits. Many could provide no explanation, other than habit and taste, for their choices of food, even when asked to look back and consider how they originally made their choice. In the framework of Prochaska and DiClemente (1984), most individuals are in the pre-contemplation stage in relation to any significant behavioural change; they are not actively seeking information to guide intended behavioural changes. Even when rational consideration is given to a behaviour, this may occur after the event. Ingham and van Zessen (1997), for example, found that 36 per cent of a sample of young persons reported that they frequently considered the risks associated with unsafe sex, but did so only after the event. For this group, such consideration appeared not so much a rational assessment of potential danger, but a way of coping with (and perhaps rationalizing away) perceived risk.

With these findings in mind, Hunt and Martin (1988) suggest that the first objective of any attempt at behavioural change should involve breaking the routine of already established behaviours. Such changes need not be complex, and may involve simple environmental changes such as small alterations to the layout of foods in a supermarket or not putting ashtrays on tables in restaurants. According to Hunt and Martin, such changes need not necessarily identify alternative behavioural choices. The act of interrupting a routine behaviour and forcing cognitive work may, in itself, be sufficient to facilitate appropriate behavioural change. This approach differs from the provision of prompts to behavioural change such as signs or advertising, as these do not interrupt behaviour and, accordingly, may be less likely to facilitate cognitive processing. Nevertheless, the two approaches may work synergistically to promote change.

Whose rationality?

A central assumption of many of the models reviewed is that we work on the basis of rationality, and that this is governed by a common desire to preserve health. However, behaviour may be guided by other 'rationalities'. Both Graham (1976) and Jacobson (1981), for example, found that many working-class women smokers made a 'rational' choice to use smoking as a means of controlling the stresses of coping with adverse social and material circumstances, in the full knowledge of its long-term health-damaging effects. Many reported that, in the context of their life circumstances, the time and effort required to quit were not available or afforded high priority.

Again using the example of smoking, Ingham and Bennett (1990) suggest that the very threat to health carried on all cigarette packets may serve to encourage or maintain smoking in social worlds in which risk-taking is a highly valued means to advancement. This form of alternative rationality can be used also to explain why some people do not use condoms despite their understanding of their protective value. Both Pivnick (1993) and Sobo (1993), for example, interviewed a number of HIV positive women about their use of condoms, many of whom did not use a condom with their lover or husband, but did so with more casual sexual partners. For them, the lack of a condom implied commitment to a long-term relationship, and a desire to become as intimately involved as possible only within that relationship. This risky behaviour was viewed as strengthening the relationship between them and their partner. Conversely, the use of condoms implied a casual, non-committed, relationship. Here, the use of a condom carried a strong rationality and a shared meaning between partners beyond its health-protective value.

Social and familial determinants of behaviour

Behaviours do not take place in a social or cultural vacuum, and many behaviours carry meanings beyond the simple behavioural act. Dorn (1983), for example, reported how youthful drinking behaviour is frequently culturally determined. Forms of drink buying, particularly 'round buying', were seen by those involved as part of the group's collective response to the material conditions in which it is situated. It demonstrated the independence and equality of individuals, while enabling reciprocal public exchange. Here, control of consumption is taken by the group, and typically rises in comparison with the amount drunk alone or in the company of one other person. This culture may also insulate young people from traditional health promotion programmes which are of little relevance to them as individuals and are likely to be strongly countered by the demands of their social group

Family processes also impact significantly on a number of health-related behaviours (see Chapter 8, pages 134–7). Many women still control the content of individual meals, although families' overall diet is often a negotiated compromise between the choices of differing family factions (Backett 1990). A final example stems from work in the negotiation, or otherwise, of sexual relationships. Here, there is consistent evidence that women, and in particular young women, are relatively disempowered in such negotiations, and the choice of whether or not to use a condom or engage in other safer sex practices is frequently made by the male partner (Holland *et al.* 1990).

Summary and conclusions

Social cognition models, such as those described above, provide a parsimonious understanding of the cognitive processes involved in behavioural decision-making. Behaviour is considered consequent to a complex process involving consideration of attitudes, cost–benefit analyses, and outcome and efficacy judgements. While the emphasis of the models is on cognitive factors, social and environmental processes are also considered in the form of social norms, barriers to change and in Ajzen's dimension of control over behaviour. Accordingly, the models provide a rationale for health promotion initiatives or policies targeted both at the individual and their wider environment. However, it is important that the models are not used in a restrictive manner. Effective use of the models requires moving significantly beyond the individual and considering their implications for social, environmental, and public health policies (see Part III). In addition, other research methodologies may provide important insights into the processes involved in the adoption of health behaviours, which the relatively constrained (questionnaire-based) methodologies used in social cognitive research cannot. Here we are thinking of qualitative and ethnographic methods in particular. Individually, the models we have described only explain between 20 and 30 per cent of the variance in health behaviours; we still have some way to go before we achieve a fuller understanding of these processes. A pluralistic approach may bring this nearer to fruition.

Suggested reading

Bennett, P. and Hodgson, R. (1992) Psychology and health promotion. In G. Macdonald and R. Bunton (eds) *Health Promotion: Disciplines and Diversity*. London: Routledge.

Bennett, P., Murphy, S. and Carroll, D. (1994) Social cognition models as a framework for health promotion: necessary, but not sufficient. *Health Care Analysis*, 3: 15–22.

Conner, M. and Norman, P. (eds) (1996) *Predicting Health Behaviour: Research and Practice with Social Cognition Models*. Buckingham: Open University Press.

PART

II

Facilitating individual change

Influencing health behaviour: individual change

Effective health promotion initiatives employ a variety of methods to facilitate behavioural change. Many are targeted at whole populations, or large subgroups such as gay men, smokers, and so on. These frequently employ methods of mass communication, legislation, or environmental change. Others may target individuals using one-to-one, or group, educational or counselling methods. Each approach has advantages and disadvantages. Behavioural changes consequent to population initiatives may be relatively small and have little impact on a particular individual's risk for disease, but because of the large numbers of people involved may impact on population levels of disease. Conversely, one-to-one or group interventions may significantly reduce individual levels of risk for disease but, because of the small numbers affected, have minimal impact on population levels of disease. Accordingly, population approaches may be considered cost-effective, while individual interventions are outcome-effective. Perhaps the optimal approach is to combine the two methods, targeting high risk individuals with individual counselling while exposing the broader population to media and environmental manipulations. The Stanford heart disease prevention projects (Maccoby 1988), for example, used this approach to good effect by providing individual counselling for those at the highest risk for CHD at the same time as influencing behaviours within the wider community through media and environmental initiatives. The impact of individual counselling was further enhanced by the dissemination of relevant information to family and friends by those who were counselled, cascading information through to the larger population.

Individualized interventions gain their advantages in a number of ways. They can identify the individual's understanding of the issue in question and permit provision of information appropriate to their knowledge level. In addition, they allow issues directly pertinent to the individual to be addressed, while any resistances to change can be identified and worked through. Finally, this type of approach can provide immediate and relevant help in overcoming obstacles to change, training in any skills necessary, and support during this process.

This chapter will examine a number of ways through which individual behavioural change can be facilitated using methods appropriate to how prepared the individual is to consider change, the personal resources they have to engage in and maintain change, and the complexity of the change required. Each will be examined within a stage model of counselling before describing two particular examples of specialist counselling involving smoking cessation methods and stress management. The effectiveness of these strategies is considered in the following chapter.

A stage model of counselling

Much of our behaviour is habitual, and individuals consider or make significant lifestyle changes relatively infrequently. Even when faced with the possible benefits of behavioural change, individuals will explore such a possibility from differing perspectives and there is clear evidence that knowledge of health risk conferred by any behaviour will only motivate a certain percentage of individuals to make appropriate changes. To treat all individuals as a homogenous group with equal motivation to change their behaviour, and for whom all types of counselling will work equally, is inappropriate. The 'stages of change' model of Prochaska and DiClemente (1984; see Chapter 2, this volume) provides some indication of the interventions appropriate to different levels of motivation to change.

Prochaska and DiClemente identified five stages of behavioural change: pre-contemplation, contemplation, preparation for action, action, and maintenance or relapse. While initially intended to provide an understanding of the processes involved in change, the model has provided a number of therapeutic insights. The most important is that different strategies of counselling are relevant to different stages of the contemplation process. Exploration of how change may be achieved is a fruitless exercise for individuals who are not considering change. Similarly, attempts to increase motivation to change with someone already attempting change are likely to be less effective than consideration of how best to achieve any desired changes. What has also become clear is that direct attempts to persuade individuals to change when in the pre-contemplation stage are unlikely to foster change; indeed, they may increase resistance (Brehm and Brehm 1981; Ockene et al. 1991). A final implication of the model is that the goals of counselling necessarily differ according to the stage of change of the individual being counselled. For those in the pre-contemplation stage a successful therapeutic outcome may be a move towards more active consideration of change; for those already in the contemplation stage, the goal may be to develop action plans to promote behavioural change.

This chapter focuses on intervention approaches relevant to differing stages of change. The first section examines the process of motivating change amongst those in the pre-contemplation or contemplation stages. The next section examines issues in the provision of information during counselling relevant to these and other stages. The third section introduces the model of counselling developed by Egan (1990) relevant to those contemplating or engaged in change. The final section examines strategies and skills which may be employed or taught to facilitate specific behavioural changes, involving smoking cessation and stress management.

Motivational interviewing

Individuals in the pre-contemplation or contemplation stage rarely seek counselling. Accordingly, counselling techniques appropriate to this group have, until recently, received little consideration. However, the introduction of health screening has resulted in the identification of significant numbers of individuals who would benefit from changing their behaviour, but appear reluctant to do so. Attempts at direct persuasion appear to have little influence on this group, and the challenge for those working with them has been to develop strategies to foster change. The best approach so far seems to be that of motivational interviewing (Miller and Rollnick 1991). Initially developed for use with problem drinkers (Miller 1983), its effectiveness has now been shown with groups as diverse as smokers, people who are overweight, and those who have physical disabilities (see Rollnick et al. 1992).

The primary goal of the motivational interview is to encourage individuals to explore and attend to previously unconsidered reasons for changing their behaviour. Its practitioners argue that this process may result in a state of cognitive dissonance (Festinger 1957) in which the individual holds, and actively considers, two or more sets of opposing beliefs about a particular issue. According to cognitive dissonance theory, this is an aversive state and one which motivates cognitive or behavioural work to reduce the discomfort. This may result in a rejection of the newly considered arguments. More positively, it may result in the adoption of new beliefs or behaviours, that is, progression through the stages of change.

The role of the counsellor is to facilitate this process, not to argue in favour of change or to attempt persuasion directly (Rollnick et al. 1992). The process is deliberately non-confrontational, and hangs on two key questions: 'What are some of the good things about your present behaviour?', and 'What are the less good things about it?' Note that the potential for resistance to discussion is diffused by a tacit acknowledgement of the benefits of the behaviour in question, and that individuals are asked to consider the benefits of change only after this. Following this, a similar process may be conducted in which the individual is asked to express any concerns they may have about their present behaviour, or about change itself. The results of these discussions are then summarized and fed back to the individual by the counsellor. Only if the person then expresses some interest in change should the interview progress to providing information on change or examining ways in which this could be achieved.

Informational approaches

The simplest, and most frequent, attempt at behavioural change remains an educative process in the course of which the individual is provided with information relevant to the health behaviour requiring change. Early work suggested that such an approach can be successful, following even minimal information exchange. Russell *et al.* (1979), for example, showed that brief anti-smoking advice given by family doctors in routine consultations to all cigarette smokers attending their surgeries resulted in a 5 per cent one-year sustained cessation rate. This compared with less than 1 per cent in non-intervention controls. Much of the more recent and successful work in primary care screening programmes (e.g. OXCHECK Study Group 1994) has involved the provision of standardized information, albeit of a more complex nature, regardless of differences in the characteristics of the individual receiving the information (see Chapter 4, this volume).

While the provision of appropriate information may result in behavioural change, the results of Russell and colleagues also indicate that the effectiveness of information provision may vary markedly as a function of the person providing it. Subanalysis of the results of their study revealed that some family doctors facilitated virtually no change among the patients they advised; others achieved significantly more than the average. Clearly, some individuals are better communicators, and the way they provide information is more effective, than others.

A number of verbal and non-verbal cues and strategies facilitate good communication. One example, provides an indication of the importance of subtle aspects of communication in determining its effectiveness. Those being given the information are often reluctant to ask questions. Data from Carstairs (1970) and Mayou *et al.* (1976), for example, suggested that between half and three-quarters of the people who want more information during a medical consultation do not ask for it. Possibly as a consequence of such a failure, between 7 and 53 per cent of people report not having fully understood the information they were given, or wanting more (Ley 1988). Encouraging such questioning can significantly increase the number of questions asked during an interview and adherence to any behavioural recommendations made (Greenfield *et al.* 1985; Tabak 1988).

Ley and Llewelyn (1995) suggested further strategies to maximize recall of information and behaviour change. These strategies, based on both experimental and intervention studies, increased recall of information by between 9 and 21 per cent and improved adherence to recommended behavioural change in comparison to less structured information provision. Their guidelines included:

- stating important facts early in the information giving process;
- stressing the importance of key facts;
- using language appropriate to the individual;
- using simple words and short sentences;
- explicitly categorizing the type of information given: first listing the categories, repeating the name before each category of information is given;
- repetition;
- keeping the number 'bits' of information to the minimum required;
- giving information in summary form at the end of any interview.

An important adjunct to oral communication, and aid to recall and compliance, is the provision of written information. This has a number of advantages over oral communication. In particular, it can be consulted at any time and can be written in a format designed to maximize understanding and interest. The percentage of people who read written information is generally high when it is given in the context of an interview (Ley 1988). This contrasts strongly with the low readership of leaflets left for individuals to browse through in public places or hospitals and other health settings (Wicke *et al.* 1994).

The long-term impact of leaflets on behaviour is only modest. However, many fail to achieve even the possibility of facilitating change as a result of inadequate design. This may result from a failure to address the particular concerns of the target audience (e.g. Leathar 1981) or more technical problems such as using language that is too complex for its readership. A number of reading index scores (e.g. Flesch 1948) provide analyses of the complexity of written passages based on factors such as word length and sentence construction. These provide a score which, typically, denotes the percentage of individuals within the general population able to read a particular text. Reviews have consistently shown patient and public information leaflets to be so complex that a significant percentage of the target audience would be unable to understand the information given. Bendick and Cantu (1978), for example, estimated that the language used in 60 per cent of US welfare leaflets made them too difficult for 70 per cent of the general population to understand. As those in most need of welfare are generally the less well educated, the percentage of their target audience able to use the information provided would be considerably lower. This is not a problem of the distant past. More recent studies reveal the continued publication of many health education materials which were too difficult for their intended audience, including leaflets providing information on condom use (Richwald *et al.* 1988), mental health (Le Bas 1989) and cholesterol (Glanz and Rudd 1990).

A problem solving approach to counselling

Providing a synthesis of a both humanistic (Rogers 1967) and cognitive-behavioural approaches (e.g. Meichenbaum 1985), the counselling approach described by Egan (1990) has become one of the most widely acknowledged models of counselling. Egan identified three stages to the counselling process: problem exploration and clarification; goal-setting; and facilitating action. This logical flow is now an integral part of most cognitive-behavioural therapies, and may appear somewhat obvious. However, at the time Egan began to develop his model of therapy, unstructured and exploratory humanistic therapies formed the predominant model in counselling, and the move towards a focused, problem-based model was a marked shift of emphasis. Similarly, the model's emphasis on resolving problems in the here and now moved from the psychoanalytical approach (e.g. Freud 1967) where explanation and reduction of distress was sought through exploration and resolution of past traumas.

Egan's model is client-centred in that the primary goal of counselling is to facilitate the individual's own resources towards identifying and resolving their problems. It is not the role of the counsellor to decide what the client needs to change or to provide solutions by which such changes could be achieved. Central to his approach is the notion of self-efficacy (Bandura 1986). Without the belief that they can achieve any desired changes, the client is unlikely to engage in any attempt at change. Accordingly, the goals, and strategies by which they are to be met, need to be client-determined. Where the client does not have the resources or skills required to achieve any changes they wish to make, this can be identified and remedied through specific skills training such as assertiveness or stress management training.

Egan suggests that a key aspect of counselling is the relationship between the counsellor and their client. He suggests that counsellors must respect and empathize with their clients, express these feelings through their verbal and non-verbal behaviour, and be genuine in their counselling relationships. The counsellor must gain an understanding of the issues from the client's perspective and not be judgemental of the person. Egan also identified a number of more specific strategies for particular use at each stage of the counselling process. These are described in more detail by Egan (1990).

Stage 1: problem exploration and clarification

Here, the goal of counselling is to help the person fully understand the problems they are facing. This may sound simple, but is not necessarily so. The individual may feel so overwhelmed by a series of problems and their emotional sequelae that they are unable to identify particular issues which need resolving. They may indeed have identified the wrong issues as problematic, and a failure to progress may represent this fundamental error. Misidentification of a problem may also occur if the counsellor fails to address this phase of the counselling process appropriately, and can lead to inappropriate attempts at problem resolution (see Bennett 1993). Skills required in this phase of counselling include direct questioning, verbal prompts, and empathic feedback, through which the counsellor reflects back to the individual their understanding of the problem and feelings they are expressing.

Stage 2: goal setting

The second stage of counselling involves identifying what needs to be done to resolve the problem, defined in terms of a goal, or series of goals. Egan suggests these should be behaviourally defined, precise ('I will go to the gym twice a week', not 'I must do more exercise'), and manageable. Achievable goals can encourage change; failure reduces self-efficacy beliefs and can exacerbate the problem. At this stage, it is not necessary to identify *how* any goals will be achieved; the need is simply to clarify them. Skills and strategies involved in this stage include summarizing the problem to provide a bridge between problem identification and resolution, providing relevant information, and encouraging the individual to identify possible alternatives to the present situation.

Stage 3: facilitating action

The final stage of the counselling process involves the counsellor helping the individual to identify how the goals they have specified may be achieved, and to facilitate them through the process of change. Working out methods of achieving goals often requires consideration of a number of alternative strategies before a final approach is chosen. This may involve a process of brainstorming in which a series of possible ways of achieving the goals are identified, before active consideration is given to their merits and potential drawbacks and a final strategy chosen.

Modelling, rehearsal, and self-efficacy

The third phase of Egan's model may be particularly important in determining the effectiveness of any attempt at change or engaging in a new behaviour. As we discussed in the previous chapter, Schwarzer (1992) has suggested that an important mediator between an intention to engage in a new behaviour and its enaction is the development of action plans: thinking through how a new behaviour may be performed, what obstacles may appear, how these may be dealt with, and so on. Where the individual lacks the skills to effect any necessary behaviours, these may be taught through a process of modelling and vicarious learning. In some cases, such a process may be an informal one within a broader counselling framework. Other skills training may be a component of a more formal intervention. Many HIV prevention programmes, for example, now teach safer sex negotiation skills (O'Donnell *et al.* 1995; Weisse *et al.* 1995). Such a process may involve participants viewing a video or role playing someone effectively negotiating safer sex. The strategies and skills used are then analysed, and the individual practises their use within the safety of the group. Here, skilled behaviours are modelled, and the individual gains confidence in their use through practice combined with appropriate feedback.

Adding to the Egan model

Egan regards his model as a tool or framework to guide people through the counselling process. It is not to be used rigidly, and in reality the stages may merge and not occur in a straightforward sequence. In addition, all the stages may not be necessary for all clients, nor need they involve long periods of time. While the model allows individuals to develop a clear understanding of their problems and the changes they wish to make, some people may not have the skills or resources to do so. For this reason, Egan saw his basic framework as being able to integrate a number of adjunctive counselling and skills-based interventions. Two, particularly pertinent to health promotion, are techniques and strategies used in stopping smoking and stress management skills.

Smoking cessation skills

To develop an appropriate strategy for smoking cessation, some understanding of the processes underlying smoking are necessary. Social learning theory provides a model of many of the underlying processes. Smoking initiation is associated with exposure to cigarettes by peers and family (Hansen *et al.* 1987) who model the pleasures associated with smoking. Young people typically smoke their first cigarette in the presence of their peers and with their encouragement (Leventhal *et al.* 1985). In addition, smokers frequently associate smoking with a number of positive attributes such as attractiveness to the opposite sex and 'rebellion' (Barton *et al.* 1982). Accordingly, the first rewards associated with smoking are primarily social.

Those who smoke more than four cigarettes are likely to become regular smokers (Leventhal and Cleary 1980). For these individuals, the determinants of their smoking change over time. In particular, the pharmacological effects of smoking gain in importance. Nicotine is a powerful drug, which influences alertness and mood and is bi-phasic in nature. Long inhalations on a cigarette induce relaxation and reduce tension: short rapid inhalations increase alertness and concentration (Jarvis 1989). Inhalation is rewarded by a perceptible affective change within seven seconds. Conversely, as a consequence of the physical dependence, smoking cessation may result in significant withdrawal symptoms for some smokers. Smoking here acts as a negative reinforcer, relieving the unpleasantness of such symptoms. While nicotine regulation is important in maintaining smoking behaviour, it is not the only process involved. Smoking may become routinely associated with a number of behaviours, such as drinking coffee, answering the telephone, and so on. Smoking may also act as a form of social interaction or as a psychological coping mechanism (Ashton and Stepney 1982).

Those giving up smoking have to contend with a number of problems, including the loss of a powerful psychological support, changing a well-established habit, and the possible onset of withdrawal symptoms. Programmes which take account of these processes, and teach skills of relapse prevention, are likely to be most effective, although success rates even for such sophisticated interventions are only modest, with typical cessation rates averaging about 40 per cent immediately at the end of a withdrawal programme, and dropping to between 25 and 30 per cent after one year (Lando *et al.* 1989; Rosenbaum and O'Shea 1992).

A technology of smoking cessation

Smoking cessation can be viewed as a special case of problem solving counselling. It involves setting goals and subgoals, identifying potential barriers to achieving these goals and strategies by which these obstacles may be overcome. The process of quitting typically follows five stages: establishing motivation, identifying smoking triggers, cutting down, stopping, and relapse prevention.

Stage 1: establishing motivation

Smokers who attend smoking cessation clinics are likely to be highly motivated to stop smoking. Such an assumption cannot be made of those attending screening clinics or in the workplace. Only about 50 per cent of smokers are likely to be in the contemplation stage at any one time, while only 15 per cent are in the action stage (Prochaska *et al.* 1988). Simply attending a screening clinic may be sufficient to shift some in the pre-contemplation stage towards change. This process may be facilitated through the use of motivational interview techniques. Here, the focus should be on the immediate gains and losses of smoking as well as the longer term health consequences, as the former may be the more powerful mediators of behaviour (see Chapter 2, page 30). Such a process may benefit both those already contemplating change as well as shift those in the pre-contemplation stage.

Stage 2: identifying smoking triggers

Effective planning involves both smoker and counsellor gaining a clear understanding of when and why the individual smokes cigarettes throughout the day – whether they are a function of habit, nicotine dependence, and so on. This information can be gained through talking the individual through a typical day or through the use of a smoking diary (see Figure 3.1), in which the smoker typically records the time each cigarette is smoked during the

Time	Strength of desire	Trigger/situation
8.00	8	Just got up
8.05	3	Fancied a second
9.00	6	Driving to work
10.00	9	Break at work
10.10	4	Had a second with friend

Figure 3.1 Example of a smoker's diary

day and what triggered them to smoke it. Once the individual becomes more aware of the triggers to their smoking, they can begin to consider strategies which will help them cope with them.

Stage 3: cutting down

The best method of cessation seems to be a compromise between gradually cutting down and total cessation. Many programmes (Leventhal and Cleary 1980) recommend a period of gradual withdrawal to a level of about 12 cigarettes a day, before complete cessation. The value of such a strategy is explained by the pharmacological process evoked by reduced smoking. For most smokers, smoking more than 12 cigarettes per day maintains their blood nicotine levels consistently above the level required to prevent withdrawal symptoms. If less than this number is smoked, blood levels of nicotine dip below the level required to prevent discomfort. Each cigarette smoked then relieves this discomfort, establishing a powerful negative reinforcement schedule. A majority of smokers who try to quit gradually fail to move beyond this stage (Cinciriprini *et al.* 1994).

Accordingly, the third stage typically involves the smoker gradually reducing the number of cigarettes they smoke to about 12 a day. A number of strategies may help the individual cut out cigarettes during this phase, and prepare them for problems to be faced after quitting. These include: avoiding triggers to smoking, identifying personalized methods of coping with triggers which cannot be avoided, and gaining support from family or friends. By the end of this stage the smoker is working towards a 'quit day', beyond which they stop smoking completely.

Stage 4: stopping

Stage 4 involves achieving abstinence. About half of those who reach this point and initially quit smoking experience some degree of physical discomfort and strong cravings for a cigarette as a consequence of nicotine withdrawal. These 'symptoms' may last for up to two weeks, although they are most severe in the first two to three days after cessation. Their severity may differ markedly over several cessation attempts, and most smokers over-estimate their likely severity (Tate *et al.* 1991). Smokers who are highly nico-tine dependent may benefit from the use of nicotine substitutes at this stage; those whose smoking is predominantly habitual will benefit less (Hall *et al.* 1985). Those who wish may benefit from their occasional use before quitting, to gain experience and confidence in their use following cessation. Depend-ence can be gauged by formal assessment through questionnaires (e.g. Fagerstrom 1982), from client report or diary records of triggers to smoking.

Continued use of any strategies found helpful during the cutting down phase may also help both nicotine dependent and habitual smokers cope with the problems faced following cessation. In addition, personalized methods of dealing with cravings may be helpful. One method we have found particu-larly helpful is to maintain a positive mental set, and to reframe withdrawal symptoms as 'signs of recovery'. Other strategies can be devised through collaboration between counsellor and client.

Stage 5: relapse prevention

In order to prevent resumption of smoking (which may occur days, weeks, or even years following cessation) many programmes prepare ex-smokers to cope with future cravings and temptations. Interventions to prevent relapse include booster sessions and extended contracts, extended interventions to provide social support or to deal with some of the negative sequelae to smoking cessation, such as weight gain, or relapse prevention training skills (Marlatt and Gordon 1980). The main components of the latter include anticipating and considering methods of resisting relapse in high-risk situ-ations, and cognitive restructuring (see below) to deal with self-defeating attributions ('I've had one cigarette – that's it now, I'm back to smoking') following isolated lapses. While such interventions may benefit some smokers, these additions to smoking cessation interventions have often proven dis-appointing in their effectiveness (e.g. Minneker-Hugel *et al.* 1992).

Stress management training

Stress management procedures may be seen as an extension of the problem solving process of Egan, in that they involve identification of specific prob-lems and strategies by which these may be remedied. Stress management skills may be helpful in decreasing distress; they may also reduce risk for dis-ease. An understanding of the processes underlying stress provides a rationale for the techniques which may be used to ameliorate its effects.

The initiator of the stress response is usually an environmental event which triggers a series of psychological processes, usually in close temporal proxim-ity to this trigger event. The first of these involves a cognitive appraisal of the event. According to Lazarus and Folkman (1984), it is assessed in terms of its threat potential and the individual's perceived ability to cope with the threat. Where the threat potential of an event is high and the perceived ability to cope with it is low, the individual will experience the event as stressful. Others, such as Beck (1976), talk in more general terms of 'stressogenic' cognitions; that is, thoughts that are unrealistic and distort reality in a way which increases the perception of stress associated with the event. In both cases, cognitive content is directly associated with emotional states such as anger, anxiety and depression. Stress-engendering cognitions may also increase physiological arousal mediated by the sympathetically mediated nervous system. At low levels of stress, this is usually evidenced through increased muscular tension. Higher levels of arousal may result in a wide constellation of symptoms, including severe palpitations, sweating, and shaking. A final outcome of the stress process involves engaging in 'stressed' behaviours, including avoidance of feared situations, agitation, loss of temper, use of alcohol or drugs to reduce the experience of stress, and so on.

Each of these processes and outcomes form the target of stress management procedures. Triggers may be identified and modified using problem-focused counselling strategies, cognitive distortions through a number of cognitive techniques some of which are described below, high levels of muscular tension through relaxation techniques, and 'stressed' behaviours through consideration and rehearsal of alternative behavioural responses. Relaxation techniques are probably the most widely taught techniques in stress management programmes. Accordingly, we describe methods of learning and applying relaxation techniques in some detail. Cognitive strategies can be more complex to teach and use, and are less widely used. However, because of their centrality to the stress process, we also describe some cognitive techniques, albeit in less detail (but see Meichenbaum 1985). For an excellent introduction to a variety of easily accessible stress management strategies the reader is recommended a text by Schaefer (1987).

Relaxation training

Unlike meditation, where the goal is to provide a period of deep relaxation and 'time out', the goal of teaching relaxation skills is to enable the individual to relax as much as is possible and appropriate throughout the day, and at times of particular stress. This can both reduce levels of physical tension and other symptoms of sympathetic overarousal. Learning and using relaxation techniques may also increase perceived control over stress – itself a powerful therapeutic outcome. They are best learned through three phases: learning relaxation skills, monitoring tension in daily life, and then using relaxation at times of stress (or *in vivo* relaxation).

Learning relaxation skills

This typically involves learning relaxation under optimal conditions. Ideally, the individual is led through the process of relaxation by a trained counsellor

```
MONDAY

Time      Tension (0–10)      Trigger/situation
10.00     3                   Just getting on with work
11.00     7                   Boss demanding some work be done in a hurry
12.00     4                   Eased down a bit, but still rushed
13.00     4                   Rushed lunch
```

Figure 3.2   Example of a tension diary

with a comfortable chair or mat to lie on before practising at home using taped instructions under similar conditions. The relaxation process most commonly used is an adaptation of Jacobson's (1938) technique, which involves alternately tensing and relaxing muscle groups throughout the body in an ordered sequence. In order to use relaxation skills when under stress it is important that they are overlearned, so regular practice, typically at least once a day over a period of weeks, is necessary. As the individual becomes more skilled in the use of relaxation, the emphasis of practice shifts towards relaxation without prior tension, and relaxing specific muscle groups while using others to mimic the circumstances in which relaxation will be used in 'real life'. The order in which the muscles are relaxed varies, but a typical exercise may involve the following stages (the tensing procedure is described in brackets):

- hands and forearms (making a fist);
- upper arms (touching fingers to shoulder);
- shoulders and lower neck (hunching shoulders);
- back of neck (pushing back against support);
- lips (pushing them together);
- forehead (frowning);
- abdomen/chest (holding deep breath);
- abdomen (tensing stomach muscles);
- legs and feet (push heel away, pull toes to point at head, not lifting leg).

Monitoring physical tension

While learning relaxation skills, individuals can begin to monitor their levels of physical tension throughout the day (see Figure 3.2). This helps them identify how tense they are during the day (most people are quite surprised), likely triggers to tension in the future, and to consider how these may be moderated either through changing the context in which any stress arises or the use of relaxation techniques.

In vivo relaxation

After one or two weeks of monitoring tension and learning relaxation techniques, individuals can begin to gradually integrate them into their daily lives. Here, relaxation does not involve taking time out to relax fully; instead, it involves learning to monitor and reduce tension to appropriate levels while continuing to deal with the cause of the stress in other ways. Achieving this level of relaxation, when other things have to be attended to, takes time and practice to achieve. Initially, therefore, relaxation is best used at times of relatively low levels of excess tension. This consistent use of relaxation techniques can prepare the person to cope with times of greater tension; without practice, use of relaxation skills at such times may be difficult if not impossible. An alternative strategy that many find useful, and perhaps more easy to implement, involves relaxing at regular intervals (such as coffee breaks) throughout the day.

Cognitive interventions

Most theorists (e.g. Beck 1976; Meichenbaum 1985) agree that cognitive processes lie at the heart of the stress process. Central to these theories is the notion that stress arises, at least in part, from faulty cognitive processing. They suggest that we each interpret events which occur to us, and make judgements as to their cause and future implications. Stress or distress can arise when individuals fail to make rational appraisals of such events, and instead make judgements that are biased and distorted. Most relevant theories have focused on explanations of clinical anxiety or depression and will not be discussed here. Rather, we shall examine the cognitions thought to underlie Type A behaviour (see Chapter 1, pages 20–1).

'Stressogenic' cognitions

Two levels of cognitions involved in the stress process can be identified. Surface cognitions are the thoughts of which we are aware and can consciously evoke and change. A second order of cognition can also be identified. Cognitive schemata provide a template, or set of fundamental beliefs, which guide our interpretation of the world and hence our surface cognitions. We are usually unaware of such schema, although these may be accessed at times, such as during the counselling process. Price (1988) identified a number of cognitive schemata underlying Type A behaviour. She suggested that Type A men hold three fundamental beliefs: things that are valued (including affection and love) are in short supply, it is not a 'fair world', and we have to strive actively and continually to obtain things we value. In addition, Price argued that Type A men have low self-esteem and constantly strive to obtain the approval of others. As they place little value on themselves as people, they believe such approval can only be gained through achievement. As approval is in short supply and needs to be actively worked for, Type As find themselves continually trying to achieve and to prove themselves worthy of other people's regard.

Cognitive interventions

Two strategies for changing cognitions are frequently employed. The first, and simplest, was developed by Meichenbaum (1985) and is targeted at surface cognitions. Self-instruction training involves interrupting the flow of stress-provoking thoughts and replacing them with more positive or coping ones. These typically fall into one of two categories. The first category of cognitions act as reminders to use any stress coping techniques the person has at their disposal ('You're winding yourself up here – come on, calm down, deep breath'). The second form of self-instruction is more akin to reassurance, reminding the individual that they can cope effectively with the feelings of stress at the time ('Come on you've dealt with this before – you should be able to again'). To ensure relevance to the individual, and that they can actually evoke these thoughts at times of stress, Meichenbaum suggests that particular coping thoughts should be considered, wherever possible, before the stressful events occur. Their use may be planned through a process of rehearsal either within the therapy session and guided by a counsellor, or by the individual alone.

A more complex intervention involves identification and challenging the veracity of stress-engendering thoughts (Meichenbaum 1985). It asks the individual to consider such thoughts as hypotheses, not facts, and to assess their validity without bias. It may involve consideration of both surface cognitions and, also, more fundamental cognitive schemata. This rational examination of hypotheses may draw on a number of lines of evidence for consideration. One such technique involves distancing, helping the individual to see the event from the perspective of others. This is shown in the following dialogue between a Type A man, Peter, who had previously driven dangerously fast to arrive at a meeting in time, and his counsellor:

Peter: Well, I had to be at the meeting on time. I just had to be, so I drove as fast as I could.

Counsellor: What were you saying to yourself as you drove?

Peter: Well, I had a lot of angry thoughts, such as: 'Come on you %^$ get out of my way,' and 'Hurry up!!! I'm going to be late!'

Counsellor: Why was it so important for you to be at the meeting on time?

Peter: I'm not sure . . . I just hate being late.

Counsellor: Why?

Peter: I guess it's because it's a sign of weakness. If I'm late people will think I'm not doing a good job, that I'm incompetent.

Counsellor:	So keeping time is a sign of competence, which must be achieved at all times. You need people to know that you're keeping on top of things.
Peter:	Yes. I guess I want them to approve of me!
Counsellor:	How do *you* react if someone is late for a meeting?
Peter:	Well, to be honest, I don't really think anything of it – I just assume that they are busy, or they've been held up, or whatever.
Counsellor:	So, you don't judge people on being late. Why do you think they make such judgements about you, if you don't make them about them?
Peter:	Well, if you put it like that . . . Yes, well I suppose they probably don't. It's probably me worrying over nothing.

Here, Peter is encouraged to question the assumptions behind his anxieties, not simply to accept them as true. The intention of therapy would be to encourage him to engage in a similar internal dialogue when faced with a stressful situation in the future, in the hope that he would behave differently. Note that the counsellor identified a number of surface cognitions before exploring and attempting to modify deeper cognitive schemata. These and other cognitive techniques are described in more detail in Meichenbaum (1985).

Summary and conclusions

This chapter has focused on methods of facilitating change in one-to-one (or group) counselling. Such interventions are relatively time consuming, and from a health promotion perspective outcome-effective, rather than cost-effective. For maximum effect, the form of the intervention must be congruent with the stage of change of the individual involved. Where the individual is not considering change, the goal of any intervention may only be to progress them along the change continuum towards consideration of change. For those in the contemplation or action stages, the goal of any intervention should be to facilitate change. Some individuals may be able to achieve this following the provision of appropriate information. Others, who perhaps face more complex problems in achieving change or are less confident in their ability to do so, may require further counselling. A problem-solving approach, in which the goal of the counsellor is to facilitate the coping skills of the individual, may be the most appropriate intervention here. Finally, where the individual needs new skills in order to achieve change, these may be taught in either a one-to-one or a group setting. In the following chapter we examine where these approaches have been used to facilitate changes in a number of health-related behaviours and to examine their effectiveness in doing so.

Suggested reading

Bennett, P. (1993) *Counselling for Heart Disease*. Leicester: British Psychological Society.

Egan, G. (1990) *The Skilled Helper. Models, Skills, and Methods for Effective Helping*. Monterey, CA: Brooks Cole.

Meichenbaum, D. (1985) *Stress Inoculation Training*. New York: Pergamon.

Schaefer, W. (1987) *Stress Management for Wellness*. New York: Holt, Rhinehart & Winston.

Individually targeted interventions

CHAPTER 4

Although many programmes designed to facilitate behavioural change are established in the communities in which people live or the worksites where they are employed, many fail to utilize these environments in ways which could enhance the process of change. Nevertheless, programmes targeted at individual behavioural change are increasingly common and, as a consequence of their lack of contextual integration, relatively easy to initiate and maintain. In this chapter we examine the effectiveness of three types of these interventions: self-help approaches, screening and educational interventions, and more complex counselling. The literature relevant to each of these areas is substantial and beyond the scope of this chapter to cover in depth. Accordingly, we focus here on representative studies rather than attempting a complete review of the relevant literature.

Bibliotherapy and self-help manuals

Perhaps the simplest method of facilitating behavioural change is through the provision of information leaflets. Evidence of their effectiveness is mixed. In a comprehensive and influential review, Gatherer *et al.* (1979) concluded that leaflets often produce limited and short-lived changes in knowledge and behaviour. More recent evidence supports their conclusions, with evidence that their use may result in increased knowledge (Roland and Dixon 1989; Brook and Smith 1991) and, in some cases, appropriate behavioural change (Russell *et al.* 1979). However, any gains are frequently lost over time (Cole and Holland 1980; Metson *et al.* 1991).

While the content of a leaflet has clear implications for its effectiveness (see Chapter 3, this volume), so too do the context and process of its use. Significant changes in recall, knowledge and behaviour are most likely when a leaflet is used in conjunction with counselling (e.g. Russell *et al.* 1979), other educational resources (McMaster *et al.* 1985), comes from a reliable source (Ley *et al.* 1976), or is used within a familiar context (Roland and Dixon 1989). Less successful outcomes are associated with unsolicited mail drops and leaflets unsupported by a health professional (Gatherer *et al.* 1979). The use of posters and waiting room notice boards has similarly been criticized as ineffective. Wicke *et al.* (1994), for example, asked a sample of 600 patients who had used a UK family doctor's waiting room to recall health messages on its public notice board. Less than a quarter recalled any topic correctly and less than 10 per cent had read or taken a health promotion leaflet related to the topics on display. Of interest is that many health professionals doubt the efficacy of leaflets. Murphy and Smith (1993), for example, found that a majority of health professionals who regularly used leaflets, such as community pharmacists and health visitors, were unconvinced of their ability to increase knowledge or change behaviour. In addition, many questioned whether the leaflets were read by those to whom they were given.

Self-help materials allow more complex information to be given than leaflets. They can provide substantial information and even, in some cases, a structured approach to achieving change. Klesges *et al.* (1989) reported that, on average, 31 per cent of smokers quit smoking after their use of self-help materials. Long-term abstinence rates of 26 per cent also compared favourably with more intensive interventions. However, the results of such interventions are extremely variable. Decker and Evans (1989) found a 'by mail' smoking cessation course to be as effective as a series of five weekly meetings combined with a telephone hot-line, reporting one-year follow-up abstinence rates of 37 and 41 per cent respectively. By contrast, Owen *et al.* (1989) compared the effectiveness of a number of sophisticated smoking cessation correspondence courses with a control intervention comprising brief information on smoking cessation. Immediately following the courses, participants who were involved in the correspondence courses reported higher levels of abstinence than those in a control group. However, these gains were no longer evident at three and nine-month follow-up assessments.

Perhaps the most ambitious programme using self-help materials was reported by Fries *et al.* (1992). They reported a study in which 103,937 individuals were enrolled in a health programme provided by their insurance company (Blue Cross and Blue Shield). Enrolment occurred over a period of five years and individuals were assessed every six months after enrolment. Each participant was invited by letter to participate in the programme and asked to complete a simple health status questionnaire. Based on these reports, participants were sent individual programmes which identified future health goals and how these could be achieved. The complexity of the language and information given differed according to the educational background of the individual participants. At each six-month assessment, participants' risk scores were compared with those of new enrolees to the programme during the preceding six-month period, permitting a comparison between the effects of the programme and trends in the wider population.

These comparisons revealed significant reductions in risk for CHD among participants but not the general population. For those under 65 years, reductions in the number of cigarette smokers (–12 per cent), serum cholesterol (–4.6 per cent), alcohol consumption (–12 per cent) and an increase in the numbers of those exercising (6 per cent) were found. General population changes during this period reflected no overall trends on any of these measures. These data suggest that self-help programmes may prove an important means of improving population levels of health. However, the potentially coercive nature of a health programme provided by the insurance company which insured participants' own health suggests that these results need replication in other populations before they can be considered widely applicable.

Screening programmes

The last decade has been associated with a substantial shift of resources towards primary care and the prevention of disease in many western countries. Perhaps the most obvious manifestation of this movement has been the establishment of screening clinics to which individuals are invited, assessed for risk factors associated with a number of diseases, and advised about preventive action should this be necessary. Some programmes, such as those involving cervical screening, may lead to medical intervention should risk factors be identified. Others, particularly those targeted at risk factors associated with CHD, may require individual behaviour change to reduce risk for disease. Perhaps the most controversial screening programmes are those which identify risk for genetic disorders, such as for the gene carrying risk for cystic fibrosis (Payne et al. 1992), which may require individuals to make behavioural decisions potentially affecting future generations' health.

While the impact of screening on any one individual's health is likely to be only modest, because of the large number of people involved screening programmes may substantially affect population rates of disease. However, it should also be noted that screening clinics are most likely to be attended by white-collar, educated individuals who are already engaging in many health-promoting behaviours; those most at risk for disease attend least frequently (Greenland et al. 1992).

For those that do attend, one would predict that the change is most likely where the problem was previously unrecognized and change is easy. Here, the individual is exposed to a new threat and a cost–benefit analysis likely to favour change. Accordingly, information on serum cholesterol level may impact more than advice to quit smoking. Although comparisons between studies which examine different outcomes is not without problems of interpretation, the data would seem to support this hypothesis.

One of the largest trials measuring the effectiveness of a one-off screening process was reported by the Imperial Cancer Research Fund OXCHECK Study Group (1994). They randomly allocated a population of over 5000 adults to either a screening health check or a no intervention control condition. The health check was conducted by nurses, who assessed risk for CHD using measures including dietary fat intake, exercise and smoking levels, and blood pressure and then advised on any necessary behavioural change.

Evaluation of the project involved comparisons of participants' risk factor assessments two or three years following their health checks with those of people attending their initial health check at the same time. Overall, participants who had received the health check evidenced a 2.3 per cent lower serum cholesterol level than those in the comparison group and blood pressure measurements were lower by 2.5 per cent. However, the differences in cholesterol levels were significant for women but not men, and no differences on measures of smoking or body mass index were found. Whether any greater changes would have been found closer to the time of the health check can only be speculated upon, but the evidence of this study suggests that screening may only promote minimal long-term behavioural change.

Some evidence to suggest that screening may impact more in the short term is provided by Redman et al. (1995). Their study was based in a primary care setting, and measured the effectiveness of random screening and information provision for individuals found to have high serum cholesterol levels. The intervention comprised either feedback of cholesterol level and provision of brief written material or a longer educative period (five minutes on average) combined with additional written information. At four-month follow-up, serum cholesterol levels had fallen substantially: in the feedback condition by 0.5 mmol/litre and by 0.84 mmol/litre in the intervention group. Whether or not the advantage gained in the latter group was from the increased period of contact with the doctor or from the more comprehensive literature provided is not clear. However, the failure of a British study (Neil et al. 1995) to find any differences in effectiveness between advice on cholesterol reduction given by a dietitian, nurse, or through written materials suggests that even relatively basic dietary information combined with knowledge of risk may be sufficient to engender behavioural change.

The failure of the OXCHECK intervention to modify smoking has been replicated in a number of smaller studies (e.g. Rose et al. 1980; Li et al. 1984). These studies contrast with the early work of Russell et al. (1979) who found modest but significant cessation levels following screening and brief advice to quit. This change in the effectiveness of screening interventions perhaps reflects changing public perceptions of the health risks of smoking cigarettes and significant reductions in smoking levels within the population (OPCS 1988). It may be that those who can give up smoking without substantial help have now done so, leaving a group of smokers, many of whom wish to quit, but who have found it impossible to do so. Similarly, while some studies have found screening to reduce alcohol consumption in heavy drinking men (Anderson and Scott 1992), these results have not always been replicated in women (Scott and Anderson 1991) or in mixed populations (Heather et al. 1987; Richmond et al. 1995).

Screening interventions followed by some form of follow-up counselling may be more effective. Another large British trial of the effectiveness of screening in primary care involved over 5000 participants in 13 towns throughout mainland Britain (Family Heart Study Group 1994). Participants in the active condition received a screening procedure similar to that of the OXCHECK group. In addition, dependent on the level of risk identified, participants were offered further counselling at between two and six monthly intervals during the following year. The study design mirrored that of the OXCHECK group, with assessments comparing participants' risk factor measures at one-year post-screening with those of people attending their initial health check at the same time. In contrast to the comparison group, participants' levels of cigarette smoking were lower by 4 per cent, average blood pressures by five mmHg, weight by one kilogram, and serum cholesterol by 0.1 mmol/litre (4 per cent). This resulted in differences of risk scores for CHD averaging 12 per cent between the groups. These differences were greater than reported by the OXCHECK group (albeit measured closer to the time of screening), suggesting that additional counselling may promote greater behavioural change than screening alone.

More specific and controlled studies have also evidenced the additional benefits conferred by combining screening with follow-up counselling. Rose *et al.* (1980) found 12 per cent abstinence rates at five-year follow-up in a group of employees at high risk for CHD following four consultations by company physicians. This compared with no reduction in smoking level among those at similar levels of risk who only received screening. Among all participants in the programme, the results were more modest, although still favouring the more prolonged intervention. Seven per cent of all those participating in the extended programme had quit smoking, in comparison to none who only received one screening interview. In the context of a worksite screening programme, Blair and colleagues (1986) compared the effectiveness of screening plus advice alone or in combination with follow-up group meetings on exercise levels. Participants in the combined intervention evidenced an increase in energy expenditure during vigorous activity of 104 per cent in comparison with a 33 per cent increase among those receiving screening only. In addition, Fielding *et al.* (1995) compared the impact of a screening and a one-off advice session with screening followed by brief monthly sessions focusing on change goals for reducing serum cholesterol levels. A significantly greater proportion of those in the extended intervention group reduced their cholesterol level below that of risk for CHD.

The evidence suggests that counselling in addition to the initial screening does contribute to promoting and maintaining behavioural change. However, the mechanisms through which these gains are achieved are unclear. Additional counselling may help individuals explore more effectively how they can achieve change, and provide an opportunity for them to discuss any problems they have experienced with a person who can help their resolution. They may simply act as reminders of the need to change, or 'cues to action'.

These issues, and the cost-effectiveness of the more extended interventions, form some of the questions for the next generation of research into the effectiveness of screening. What is clear, however, is that screening is not a neutral process. While it may facilitate behavioural change it may also have a number of less positive consequences.

Early evidence that adverse health information may give rise to substantial levels of anxiety and lower perceived health was reported by Haynes *et al.* (1978). They found that individuals identified as having high blood pressure following a worksite screening programme were more anxious about their health and had twice as many days off over the following year as in the year prior to screening. Even where no risk for disease is found, health anxieties may be raised. In a British study of the impact of screening for raised serum cholesterol, Stoate (1989) reported that levels of anxiety rose among a significant number of participants following screening even when they were told they carried no risk for CHD. False positives, where individuals are told they may be at risk and on further testing are found not to be so, also carry high levels of psychological morbidity. Lerman *et al.* (1991), for example, found that three months after mammography screening, 41 per cent of women with a benign lesion continued to worry about breast cancer, while 25 per cent reported more widespread emotional problems.

How the screening process and provision of 'bad news' is conducted appears to be an important determinant of the psychological outcome. Sensitive provision of risk information, highlighting the positive effects of risk detection, and providing sufficient information on how to reduce risk may significantly reduce its aversive impact (Rudd *et al.* 1986; Wilkinson *et al.* 1990). However, even this simple process seems beyond many programmes. In a review of the area, Marteau (1994) suggested that between 25 and 71 per cent of screening programmes advised people 'not to worry' or gave no specific advice on how to ameliorate risks when these were detected.

More complex interventions

The evidence so far considered suggests that information on potential health risk is less effective in promoting behavioural change than information combined with some form of counselling, even when this is relatively brief. This should come as no surprise. A central tenet of the social cognition models discussed in Chapter 2 is that behavioural change is mediated by a variety of processes. Frequently more important than the provision of information on risk, or how to reduce risk, are factors influencing the individual's motivation to change and their perceived or actual ability to do so. In addition, both Egan from a counselling perspective, and Schwarzer from a social cognition framework, suggest that developing plans on *how* to change contributes significantly to effective change. Modelling and practising new behaviours, as suggested by social learning theory, within a counselling framework may also facilitate appropriate change. These processes may enhance skills and modify participants' confidence in their ability to effect change. The next section examines the effectiveness of interventions which attempt to incorporate these processes, making comparisons with educational programmes where such evidence exists.

Preventing HIV transmission

'Safe sex doesn't mean no sex, it just means use your imagination' (Bragg and Marr 1991). This comment perhaps reflects the population response to the threat of AIDS. For most, the practice of celibacy is not an option. Accordingly, health promotion initiatives have attempted to encourage safer sex practices rather than the avoidance of sex. Much work remains to be done. In a sample of North American heterosexual students, for example, Hawkins et al. (1995) reported that the most frequent 'safer sex' behaviour was the use of the contraceptive pill. The least frequent sexual practice, reported by 24 per cent of the sample, was the use of condoms or dental dams. These data, gathered after more than a decade of knowledge of the risks of unsafe sex, provide strong evidence that encouraging changes in sexual practice has not proven easy.

The low prevalence of safer sex practices may still, in part, be attributable to a lack of knowledge. Wenger et al. (1995), for example, asked students and attenders at a sexually transmitted disease clinic about their last sexual behaviour and whether they considered this to have involved safer sex practices. Fifty-three per cent who considered themselves to have used safer sex practices reported having vaginal or anal intercourse without using a condom during that encounter. Clearly, there remains a role for public education in preventing the spread of AIDS. However, although such an approach may increase knowledge about safer sex practices (DiClemente et al. 1987), evidence that information alone is sufficient to change behaviour is lacking (Bellingham and Gillies 1993; St Lawrence et al. 1995).

Skills-based or problem-solving interventions seem more effective. Kelly et al. (1994), for example, compared a five-session skills-based programme with an education-only control group in a group of socially disadvantaged sexually active women considered to be at high risk for HIV infection. The intervention included risk education, training in condom use, practising sexual assertiveness, problem-solving and risk trigger self-management. At the three-month follow-up, women from both conditions reported having a similar number of sexual partners. However, what they did with those partners differed; women in the intervention group reported that more of their partners used condoms, and on more occasions.

Complex interventions may impact on groups frequently considered resistant to health promotion messages. Malow et al. (1994), for example, compared the effectiveness of a skills-based and an information programme with hard drug users. The skills-based intervention comprised a series of small group meetings, totalling six hours, designed to enhance knowledge and attitudes regarding HIV prevention, improve skills in condom use and needle sterilization, and to modify high-risk sexual and drug-related behaviours. Following intervention, participants in this group reported greater self-efficacy, condom use skills, and sexual communication skills than those in the comparison group. In addition, they reported significantly greater reductions on a number of measures of sexual HIV-risk behaviour than those in the information-only condition.

One particularly powerful method of changing behaviour is through the use of videos. These permit ways of handling conflict, embarrassment, and stress surrounding the potentially awkward social transactions required in sexual risk reduction to be modelled. Kolata (1987) reported a study involving gay men, in which participants discussed issues relating to safer sex following either provision of written materials or watching an erotic safer sex video. Those in the latter group evidenced increased use of safer sex practices in comparison with those who received only written materials. O'Donnell et al. (1995) compared the effectiveness of video-based interventions designed to promote safer sex among African-American and Hispanic attenders at a sexually transmitted disease clinic in South Bronx, New York. Attenders were randomly allocated to one of three groups: no treatment control, video, or video plus interactive group 'skill-building session'. This comprised a 20-minute meeting in which barriers to condom use were identified and addressed through the provision of information, discussing condom options, and practising condom negotiation skills. All those participating in the study were provided with coupons redeemable for free condoms at a local pharmacy. In comparison to the control condition, those who saw the video were more likely to redeem condom coupons (21 versus 28 per cent). Participation in the interactive sessions further increased redemption rates to 40 per cent.

In a more radical study, Robert and Rosser (1990) compared the effectiveness of four interventions aiming to reduce unsafe sex practices in a sample of gay men. Each was randomly assigned to one of four conditions. The first involved watching a 15-minute video on AIDS, which provided information on and modelled a number of safer sex behaviours, including placing a condom on an erect penis and refusing to participate in unsafe sexual behaviour. The second condition involved 20 to 30 minutes of individual counselling in which major sexual concerns were discussed and standardized information on safer sex given. A third condition involved attendance at a workshop which explored how to eroticize safer sex practices. The final intervention involved attending a workshop in which the social impact of HIV/AIDS and safer sex guidelines were discussed. Trend analysis revealed that individual counselling was most effective in increasing condom use, while the erotic safer sex group was the only condition to evidence a significant reduction in the frequency of anal intercourse. Of interest was the finding that the conditions which engaged individuals in active consideration of how to change their behaviour evidenced the greatest behavioural change, and that these changes reflected the topics discussed. That is, each intervention may have produced effects specific to the issues addressed within it.

Such specificity of outcome was also reported by Weisse *et al.* (1995). In their study, a group of young adults took part in an AIDS prevention workshop aimed at reducing embarrassment while purchasing condoms, and encouraging their use. Half this group then participated in an exercise involving the purchase of condoms at local shops. All participants evidenced greater knowledge about AIDS and more positive attitudes towards the use of condoms immediately after the workshop, but these changes did not persist. However, those who participated in the exercise reported less embarrassment during the subsequent purchase of condoms; a change which persisted over time. The authors concluded that these results indicate that AIDS prevention workshops may lead only to transient changes unless specific skills are considered and practised.

While problem-solving or skills-based interventions appear to be more effective than purely educational interventions, these need not be time-consuming. The Talking Sex project (Tudiver *et al.* 1992) compared the effectiveness of single and four-session discussion and skills-training groups with a waiting list control. Overall, both intervention groups gained more than the control group, but no substantial differences between the two types of intervention were found; if anything, any differences favoured the one-off group meetings. In addition, such interventions need not be conducted in formal settings. Blakey and Frankland (1995), for example, reported an intervention involving outreach contact with prostitutes in a Welsh city. Over a four-year period, a worker informally met prostitutes on the streets. On each occasion, she provided information about the prevention of HIV infection and other health matters, as well as providing condoms. In addition, she discussed strategies by which the women may be able to encourage safer sex with clients who asked for unprotected sex. Over the period of the intervention, the women reported increased use of condoms and safer drug use through needle exchange and reduced needle sharing. A third of the women also passed on HIV prevention information, including leaflets and comics with HIV prevention messages, to their clients. Such results suggest that long-term programmes working in the context of the individuals involved may prove highly effective. Working within such contexts also permits the use of existing social networks as a resource. Quirk *et al.* (1993), for example, found peer education was more effective in increasing knowledge about safe intravenous drug use than formal health care workers.

Reducing risk for coronary heart disease

A number of apparently disparate behaviours contribute to risk for CHD. The screening interventions so far described have attempted to identify any, or all, of the key risks carried by those who are screened and to help change them in some way. A number of more complex interventions have had the same goal. More, however, have targeted specific risk factors. In this section, we examine interventions targeted at a broad spectrum of risk behaviours before focusing on the research literature relevant to two single-risk factor interventions: reducing blood pressure and smoking.

Multi-factorial studies

In contrast to most screening programmes in primary care settings, Gomel *et al.* (1993) reported a project in which participants took part in a substantial counselling process. In this study, over 400 workers at various Australian worksites identified through screening as having some risk factors for CHD were randomly allocated to one of three conditions: no treatment control, risk factor education, or behavioural counselling. Participants in the risk factor education group were provided with standard advice on the lifestyle changes required to reduce risk for heart disease. They were also provided with an educational resource manual and videotapes containing information on how to modify risk factors for heart disease. Behavioural counselling involved participants in up to six lifestyle counselling sessions over a 10-week period. A self-instructional lifestyle change manual containing programmes for modifying major risk factors was also provided. The behavioural counselling and manual were based on Prochaska and DiClemente's (1984) model of change. In the preparation stage, reasons for, and barriers to, change were identified. Participants also monitored behaviours contributing to their risk for CHD and identified high-risk situations and coping strategies for dealing with them. In the action stage, short and long-term goals for risk factor change were determined and strategies for achieving them considered. In the following stages, strategies for maintaining behavioural change and avoiding relapse were discussed. Participants were assessed at three, six, and 12 months following baseline assessment.

Significant differences favouring the behavioural counselling group were found on measures of blood pressure, body mass index, and percentage of body fat throughout the follow-up period. Reductions in cigarette smoking favoured the behavioural group at the three-month-follow-up, and these were maintained until the one-year assessment; seven per cent of the behavioural group had remained abstinent for one year, in comparison to none in the education-only intervention. Measures of cholesterol did not vary in any condition throughout the assessment period, while aerobic capacity in all groups initially increased but then declined. While encouraging, these outcomes were not substantially better than those obtained in the Family Heart Study (see above), and suggest that such an elaborate intervention may not be cost-effective in the primary prevention of CHD.

Behavioural change and health gain is not limited to the young and middle-aged adult population. The San Diego Medicare Preventive Health Project (Mayer *et al.* 1994) compared the effects of health risk appraisal combined with counselling and group sessions with an assessment-only condition in a group of older persons. The intervention was explicitly based on the principles of social learning theory and the Egan counselling model, and involved health appraisal, feedback, and behavioural goal setting. Two face-to-face sessions were followed by telephone contact over the following year. This was combined with an eight-week series of group meetings, exploring issues in health and ageing. By the end of the year, those in the intervention group evidenced higher levels of both stretching ability and strength, reduced fat intake, increased dietary fibre content, and a lower caffeine intake than controls.

Lowering blood pressure

Over the past decade, an increasing number of treatment trials have examined the effectiveness of diet and exercise as a means of controlling blood pressure. Stamler *et al.* (1989), for example, allocated overweight hypertension-prone individuals to either a monitoring condition or one in which they were asked to eat a low fat diet, reduce their alcohol intake to two drinks per day, and increase their exercise to three periods of 30 minutes per week. Although only a minority of participants achieved all the dietary and behavioural goals set, during the five years of the trial the incidence of hypertension was more than twice as high in a monitoring condition than in the intervention group (19.2 versus 8.8 per cent).

In a study of the effectiveness of a combined pharmacological and behavioural intervention, the Treatment of Mild Hypertension Study (Elmer *et al.* 1995) allocated mildly hypertensive persons to one of five pharmacological or placebo interventions in combination with a lifestyle intervention programme. This comprised a six-month period of intensive intervention involving both individual and group counselling sessions. These focused on modifying diet and alcohol intake and increasing levels of exercise. The intervention adopted an approach based on social learning principles. For example, participants were taught to recognize and modify cues that led to overeating, modify their attitudes towards eating, and worked with spouses to foster social and marital support for any changes made. At the one-year follow-up, all the intervention groups evidenced significant behavioural change. Seventy per cent remained below baseline weight, alcohol intake was reduced by 1.6 drinks per week, while reported leisure physical activity had increased by 86 per cent over baseline measures. These changes were associated with clinically significant reductions in diastolic (8 mmHg) and systolic (10 mmHg) blood pressure at the one-year follow-up which were maintained up to the four-year follow-up. Similar findings have been replicated in non-medicated populations (e.g. HPT Research Group 1990) and in stable medicated hypertensives (Stamler *et al.* 1986).

Affirming the multifactorial nature of hypertension, a number of studies have suggested that blood pressure may also be controlled by the use of stress management procedures, reducing the sympathetic drive thought to be involved in the development of hypertension (Obrist 1981). Many studies have reported significant reductions in blood pressure measured in the clinic following relaxation training (Bennett and Carroll 1997). Now two issues dominate the literature. First, do any changes in blood pressure found in the clinic reflect a more general reduction during everyday life? Second, do relaxation-based interventions reduce blood pressure more than other 'control' procedures?

Evidence of a generalized reduction in blood pressure stems from one of the few studies to measure pressures during participants' daily routine at their worksite (Agras *et al.* 1983). Participants were randomly allocated to either relaxation training or a no treatment control condition. Semi-automatic blood-pressure monitors were used to record their blood pressures every 20 minutes throughout the day both before and after this phase. No differences between the groups were evident before the treatment phase. However, clinically significant differences, in the order of 10 mmHg, favouring the relaxation group were found on both clinic and worksite measures following the treatment phase.

Whether relaxation is more effective than other procedures has proven a more complex question. Irvine *et al.* (1986) compared a relaxation-based intervention with a placebo control, in which participants were told that extremely gentle mobility and flexing exercises would dilate arterioles within the muscles, and (as there was now more space for the same amount of blood to occupy) reduce overall blood pressure. Participants in the active intervention evidenced significantly greater reductions in blood pressure than those in the control group immediately after the eight-week intervention period and at follow-up assessment. Accordingly, it seems that any reductions in blood pressure following learning relaxation skills cannot be attributed to placebo effects. However, relaxation appears to be no more effective than other interventions designed to reduce stress in other ways (Wadden 1984), although it is more effective than exploratory psychotherapy (Taylor *et al.* 1977). In addition, there is some evidence to suggest that cognitive therapy may enhance the effect of relaxation (Chesney *et al.* 1987), perhaps because it encourages and maintains any behavioural change.

Smoking cessation

Smoking is highly resistant to change. Once established it is maintained by addictive and conditioning processes as well as social factors. It is also an effective method of moderating stress (Shiffman 1986). This combination of factors suggests that interventions to help smokers cease smoking have to address a number of issues, and that more complex interventions may be more effective than simple exhortations to quit, even when these are combined with some minimal support.

Most intervention models now follow approaches similar to those described in Chapter 3. The American Lung Association programme, for example, has a programme involving a specific quit date, interruption of conditioned responses supporting smoking, identification and preparation of plans for coping with temptations after cessation, teaching relapse prevention skills, and follow-up contact and support. This programme, and its variants, has achieved long-term abstinence rates of between 35 and 29 per cent (Lando *et al.* 1989; Rosenbaum and O'Shea 1992).

An alternative approach to cessation involves the use of nicotine replacements. These reduce craving for cigarettes by maintaining blood nicotine levels above those required to prevent the onset of withdrawal symptoms. The first delivery method developed involved chewing nicotine gum which released nicotine to be absorbed through the mucosa. Meta-analysis suggested that nicotine gum can increase the effectiveness of cessation interventions (Lam *et al.* 1987). However, a considerable part of its effectiveness seems to lie in its placebo value (Lichtenstein and Glasgow 1992). Double-blind studies where the gum has been used in isolation have provided only mixed evidence of its effectiveness. Only when the gum has been used in combination with psychological support has its use been consistently and substantially effective (Lam *et al.* 1987). However, some failures to find this additive effect have been reported (e.g. Hall *et al.* 1987). Why this should occur is unclear. One explanation for these negative findings, however, may lie in the attributions smokers make for the success of their efforts in cessation. If success is attributed to the use of nicotine gum and not to personal coping resources, this may set up expectations of relapse when the gum is no longer used – an expectation which can become a self-fulfilling prophecy.

The equivocal success of nicotine may, at least in part, reflect the characteristics of the gum and its inappropriate use. The gum intentionally tastes unpleasant and its absorption through the mucosa can be suppressed by drinking coffee or soft drinks. Accordingly, many smokers do not use the gum sufficiently to maintain therapeutic blood levels. More acceptable, and consistent, may be the use of nicotine patches which absorb nicotine through the skin and maintain more consistent levels of plasma nicotine levels through the day. These have been shown to be more effective than a placebo (Richmond *et al.* 1994), and may enhance the impact of any behavioural intervention. Richmond *et al.* (1994), for example, compared the effectiveness of a cognitive-behavioural intervention in combination with either active or placebo nicotine patches. Participants using the active nicotine patch were most likely to be abstinent at the three (48 versus 21 percent) and six-month (33 versus 14 per cent) follow-up assessments. Six-month continuous abstinence rates were also higher among the active nicotine group (25 per cent) than the control group (12 per cent).

So far, consideration has been given to the effectiveness of smoking cessation interventions provided to all those who wish to quit smoking.

But smokers are not a homogenous group. Some smokers may smoke predominantly out of habit; some due to an addiction to nicotine (Fagerstrom 1982). Accordingly, the same therapeutic approach may not be optimal for both groups. Indeed, there is evidence that cognitive-behavioural approaches may be best for those who smoke predominantly out of habit, while nicotine replacements in combination with some form of psychological intervention may prove optimal for those with high levels of nicotine dependency. Evidence in support of this hypothesis was provided by Hall *et al*. (1985), who assigned high and low nicotine-dependent smokers to either an intensive behavioural intervention, nicotine gum, or a combination of both approaches. At the one-year follow-up, 50 per cent of high nicotine-dependent smokers in the combined intervention were not smoking. This compared with abstinence rates of 28 per cent among the equivalent group in the nicotine gum condition, and 11 per cent of those who participated in behavioural intervention. In contrast, low dependent smokers gained most from the behavioural intervention. Among this group, abstinence rates at one year were 47 per cent, in comparison to rates of 42 and 38 per cent in the nicotine gum and combined interventions.

Even where individuals have failed to quit on one attempt, it may not be unreasonable to attempt further cessation fairly quickly if the individual remains motivated to change. Gourlay *et al*. (1995), for example, randomly allocated 629 smokers who had previously failed to quit smoking while using transdermal patches to either a placebo control condition or a further intervention comprising transdermal nicotine patches, brief behavioural counselling (five to 10 minutes) and a booklet containing advice on smoking cessation and instructions for the use of patches. While quit rates were, perhaps unsurprisingly, relatively low there was still evidence of some benefit from the combined intervention, with six-month abstinence rates of 6.4 per cent of those receiving the active intervention and 3.8 per cent in the placebo condition.

The characteristics and health status of individuals entering smoking cessation programmes may be an important moderator of their success. Cessation rates are generally higher among those newly diagnosed with CHD in comparison to still disease-free populations. In addition, those at particularly high risk for disease may be more successful than others. McIlvain *et al*. (1992), for example, repeated the MRFIT smoking cessation protocol, which had previously been associated with abstinence rates of 40 per cent at the four-year follow-up in a group of men in the highest decile of risk for CHD, with a volunteer group of healthy persons. Although a high initial abstinence rate was reported (52 per cent), this had fallen to 25 per cent by the one-year follow-up – a relatively good outcome, but not comparable with the original success of the intervention.

A further factor which may powerfully influence the outcome of any intervention is the emotional state of participants. Zelman *et al*. (1992), for example, reported that 12 months following a smoking cessation course,

26 per cent of those who evidenced some degree of depression at the time of the course were abstinent. This contrasted with 62 per cent of those who were not depressed. They suggested that negative affect may have disrupted either the initial acquisition of coping skills during treatment or the generalization of those skills beyond. These findings may generalize to other populations and approaches. In a study of a community-wide stop smoking contest, Glasgow et al. (1985) also found perceived stress to be a major determinant of outcome, with those highest on measures of stress experiencing the least success in quitting.

Summary and conclusions

This chapter has provided a necessarily summary review of a substantial intervention literature. However, it highlights a dilemma faced by many of those working in public health and health promotion. More complex and sustained interventions, in general, evidence more change than short-term, information-based interventions. Those which provide counselling or support beyond a one-off risk screening interview are more effective than screening alone. In turn, more substantial and sustained behavioural changes may be consequent to complex interventions which model change or provide training in any necessary skills.

The decision of what intervention to use, and how to implement it, becomes one of cost-effectiveness and health economics. As we noted in Chapter 3, one-to-one or group interventions may significantly reduce individual participant's risk for disease but, because of the small numbers of individuals affected, have minimal impact on population levels of disease. Accordingly, population approaches may be considered cost-effective, while individual interventions are outcome-effective. Perhaps the optimal approach is to combine the two methods, targeting high-risk individuals with individual counselling while exposing the broader population to media and environmental manipulations. The final choice of intervention ultimately becomes one of economics and pragmatics rather than effectiveness.

Suggested reading

Bennett, P. and Carroll, D. (1997) Stress management approaches to the prevention of heart disease. In S. Palmer and W. Dryden (eds) Stress Management and Counselling: Theory, Practice, Research and Methodology. Cassell: London.
Fowler, G., Gray, M. and Anderson, P. (1993) Prevention in General Practice. Oxford: Oxford University Press.
Lawrence, M., Neil, A., Fowler, G. and Mant, D. (eds) (1996) Prevention of Cardiovascular Disease. An Evidence Based Approach. Oxford: Oxford University Press.
Lindsay, L. and Gaw, A. (eds) (1997) Coronary Heart Disease Prevention. A Handbook for the Health Care Team. London: Churchill Livingstone.

PART III

Facilitating population change

Environmental and public policy approaches

In a series of charter statements, the World Health Organization (WHO) has identified the need for a multilevel approach to health promotion which acknowledges the important role that the environment and public policy has on health. The first of these, the Ottawa Charter (WHO 1986), began by developing a concept of health that encompassed having social and personal resources as well as physical capabilities, and stated that health promotion should enable people to increase control over all aspects of their health. Two years later, the WHO (1988) argued that public policy should, as a priority, create environments which fostered good health. A related document (WHO 1991), identified both political and economic policy as means of enhancing the social and physical environment.

A number of strategies were identified through which the WHO's objectives could be achieved, including creating supportive environments, developing appropriate healthy public policy, increasing individuals' personal resources, and strengthening community action. Taken together, these strategies legitimize health promotion's social, political and ecological character and offer a useful framework for guiding health promotion projects focused on whole communities or societies. In this chapter we briefly expand on what the WHO meant by these strategies, before examining in more depth how they may be conceptualized in terms of psychological theory. For those interested in more critical discussion of the strategies themselves, Tonnes and Tilford (1994) provide a useful summary.

The WHO's environmental and public policy approaches

Supportive environments

The WHO called for a socio-ecological approach to health promotion, emphasizing the need to create environments supportive of health at an international, national and local level. Their approach encompassed both the need to conserve natural resources and to respond to the demands made on people by changing patterns in work, leisure, technology and urbanization. Three aspects of the environment were considered particularly relevant to health promotion. The social dimension recognized the importance of understanding and working within existing and emerging social norms, customs, and relationships when designing and implementing health promotion initiatives. The political embraced the need to increase democratic participation in decision making and to decentralize responsibilities and resources. The economic called for a rechannelling of resources into health. These strategies have led to a number of initiatives focusing on changing the physical environment to one that is more supportive of health, involving whole cities (Hancock 1993), communities within them (Farquhar *et al.* 1990), and smaller social units such as schools (Williams and de Panafieu 1985) and worksites (Maes *et al.* 1997).

Healthy public policy

In contrast to public health policy, which is a subset of policies targeted specifically at health issues, healthy public policy involves consideration of the health implications of all government policies, whatever their primary target. Using this approach, the WHO argued, governments should view health as a resource and plan to maximize its production by social and economic development across agricultural, trade, education, industrial and communication policy areas. In its most radical manifestation, this would involve central government vetting all policies for their health gain in much the same way that policies are now vetted by treasury departments (Duhl 1986; Milio 1986). Within this perspective, health promotion policy encompasses diverse but complementary approaches to improving health including legislation, taxation and organizational and environmental change. As inequalities in health arise, at least in part, from social and educational disadvantage, a number of commentators (e.g. Bunton 1992) have suggested that healthy public policy should specifically address the health and social needs of underprivileged groups.

Developing personal resources

The WHO documents emphasized the role of health promotion in helping individuals develop personal resources through the provision of information and skills training. An associated approach involves using or changing social norms to facilitate appropriate behaviour or behavioural change, or teaching resistance skills to unhealthy social norms. These manipulations may occur at the level of large communities (Puska *et al.* 1985) as well as more closely defined communities such as schools (Perry *et al.* 1986) and the workplace (Zimmerman and Connor 1989). The development of skills and, in particular, self-reliance can also be achieved through strengthening community action. This typically involves individuals or groups of individuals in identifying ways through which their community could be improved, and mobilizing resources and implementing strategies to achieve their desired goals. Communities, here, may be defined in terms of geographical proximity as well as by cultural or socio-economic similarity (Tonnes and Tilford 1994). The WHO recognized that health promotion may facilitate this process through strengthening the advocacy of groups, increasing communities' control over factors which influence health, building alliances between different groups, and mediating between interest groups.

Theoretical underpinnings

While health promotion programmes focusing on political, social and physical environments draw on materialist explanations of ill-health, they can also be linked to psychological theory. Programmes that have focused on creating supportive environments, and research highlighting the promise of healthy public policy, have been implicitly informed by social learning theory (Bandura 1977) with its emphasis on rewards and punishments and the health belief model (Becker 1974). The latter stresses the importance of facilitating behavioural change through cues to action and minimizing the costs of engaging in health-promoting behaviours, as well as increasing barriers and reducing cues to unhealthy behaviours. The processes of vicarious learning of skills and self-efficacy described by social learning theory also inform programmes involving increasing skills and personal resources.

Two further theories have implicitly informed environmental approaches, particularly those which focus on the social environment: the theory of planned behaviour (Ajzen 1985) and diffusion of innovation theory (see Rogers 1983). Both theories stress the importance of social norms as a primary influence on behaviour. Approaches to education using these theories have focused on changing inappropriate, or supporting appropriate, social norms so that the preventive behaviour becomes the norm against which individuals compare their own behaviour.

Such initiatives have not always fostered appropriate behavioural change, however, and need to be considered carefully. Ingham and Bennett (1990), for example, have suggested that at the beginning of the AIDS epidemic the heterosexual community considered the use of condoms to be a homosexual issue, irrelevant to themselves. Accordingly, uptake by the heterosexual community was much more limited than in the homosexual community where social norms became increasingly supportive of their use. These biased social norms did not simply represent prejudicial attitudes towards gays; they were actively fostered by government advertising of the time, which identified AIDS as an issue for homosexuals, intravenous drug users, and Haitians.

Creating supportive environments

Reducing barriers and increasing cues to healthy behaviour

An important form of environmental manipulation involves reducing barriers to health-promoting behaviours, and increasing cues to engage in health-enhancing behaviours. Such initiatives may occur at a national or city-wide level, for example by protecting 'green spaces' in urban areas so that they are available for recreational exercise, or through transport policies that encourage bicycle users and pedestrians over the use of cars. A more local initiative is described by Yates and Hebblethwaite (1983), in which a local public house was renovated by its patrons in order to reduce the levels of drunkenness and violence that had previously occurred there.

Product labelling, including health warnings on cigarettes and nutritional information on food, is now increasingly used as a prompt to encourage consumers to engage in health-enhancing behaviours. However, evidence of the effectiveness of such initiatives is lacking. Nutritional information on food packaging is rarely understood by the public and is used infrequently, particularly among those with low income and education (Glanz *et al.* 1995); the relatively low cost of less healthy foodstuffs may be a more salient factor than its quality for this group. Similarly, it has been found that health warnings on cigarettes are ineffective in changing existing smokers' behaviour, although they may serve to prevent the uptake of smoking (Richards *et al.* 1989).

Environmental manipulations may form isolated interventions; they may be incorporated into larger disease prevention programmes. The North Karelia Project (Puska *et al.* 1985), for example, encouraged shops and restaurants to display 'no smoking' signs, low fat sausages were produced, and the county dairy actively promoted low fat goods. In the UK, Heartbeat Wales (Nutbeam *et al.* 1993) also facilitated a number of environmental changes designed to reduce barriers and to cue appropriate behavioural change. Initiatives included encouraging food labelling and the increasing availability of healthy foods in major retailers and local butchers, facilitating the establishment of healthy restaurants (where there were identified low fat choices, no smoking areas, and so on), and providing exercise trails in local parks.

Evaluation of large-scale programmes focusing on the physical environment has proven difficult. Evaluation of the Healthy Cities movement (Hancock 1993) serves as an example. The Healthy Cities movement was a WHO-sponsored attempt to put into practice the aims and objectives of its various charters. It relied on intersectorial collaboration and community development, was concerned with positive health, and focused on ecological influences on health. Participating cities were concerned with monitoring and improving environmental indicators of quality of life including unemployment, housing quality, democratic participation and education provision

(Ashton 1992). The problem of evaluating the project was highlighted by Curtice (1991) who observed that any environmental changes were not instituted in a controlled manner and were not monitored effectively, making it impossible to establish any relationship between environmental changes and any changes in behaviour or health.

Other large-scale community programmes, such as North Karelia and Heartbeat Wales have placed great emphasis on environmental changes as a means of facilitating and maintaining appropriate behavioural change. However, these programmes typically included a number of supplementary approaches, including mass media campaigns and skills training, making it impossible to isolate the effect of environmental manipulations. The problems of isolating the effects of large-scale, and frequently ad hoc, environmental manipulations (Curtice 1991) or the specific elements of multimodal initiatives (Salonen 1987) has led to suggestions that research should place increasing emphasis on understanding the process of dissemination of programmes through communities. Nutbeam et al. (1993) argued that such measures represent legitimate health promotion outcomes in themselves as well as increasing our understanding of how any intervention influences behaviour or risk disease prevalence.

Whelan et al. (1993) identified what they termed 'intermediate outputs' as examples of such an approach. These were defined as measures of change in the social and physical environment consequent to any health promotion initiative. They include the monitoring of changes in the practice of health professionals, the development and implementation of policy statements and legislation relevant to creating health promoting environments, as well as more structural environmental changes. Examples include monitoring national and local policies to establish health promotion clinics within primary care settings and the implementation of this legislation (Kiloran 1993). Within industry, it has involved monitoring the development and implementation of health promotion policies including 'no smoking' areas or healthy food options (Eriksen 1986; Wilbur et al. 1981).

This type of approach was exemplified by the research methodology employed by the North Karelia Project (Puska et al. 1985). Intermediate outputs measured here included the number of family doctors who modified their practice to include risk factor screening clinics, how many people were screened for risk factors as a consequence, and how many shops and restaurants displayed 'no smoking' signs, or promoted low fat products. In the United Kingdom, evaluation of the Heartbeat Wales programme (Murphy and Smith 1993) similarly involved assessment of its effectiveness in encouraging food labelling, increasing access to healthy foods in major retail outlets and restaurants, and encouraging the wider distribution of low alcohol beer.

Although few in number, most controlled trials of environmental manipulation attest to their effectiveness. Studies in workplace cafés and restaurants, for example, suggest that increased availability and promotion (via posters and leaflets) of healthy foods can change knowledge and attitudes

(Wilbur *et al.* 1981) and in some cases affect behaviour (Glanz *et al.* 1995). Linegar *et al.* (1991) reported one of the few studies which has attempted to increase exercise levels within a general population through environmental manipulation. Taking advantage of the closed community provided by a naval base, they established cycle paths, exercise equipment, exercise clubs, and fitness competitions within the base. In addition, workers were given 'release time' from other duties while they participated in some physical activities. In comparison to a control area, where no such changes were initiated, significant increases in activity and fitness were found among both existing exercisers and non-exercisers in the naval base.

Closed systems, such as schools and workplaces, provide an opportunity to manipulate environmental variables and to study their impact, and both are becoming increasingly aware of the influence of appropriate health policies. A recent European initiative, for example, has utilized the potential of the school environment to foster health-enhancing behaviours. The health-promoting school programme (Williams and de Panafieu 1985) views the school as a complex social system, with all aspects of the environment exerting an influence on health. Participating schools throughout Europe are presently implementing a three-year programme involving a formal policy to maximize the promotion of good health within the school (Baric 1994). Health-related initiatives within the participating schools are not confined to an emphasis on health education. Instead, they address the interrelationship between health behaviours and encompass wider measures, including healthy nutrition and no smoking policies applicable to both pupils and teachers. These policies have resulted in the establishment of healthy food choices in canteens and smoking cessation programmes for both staff and pupils. By focusing on all aspects of school life it is hoped that educational messages are reinforced by the modelling of healthy social norms, and barriers to healthy behaviours are reduced. By the end of 1996, 36 European countries were running the initiative, all at different levels of development. They are members of a network exchanging information on implementation and disseminating good practice. Despite this, there remains a lack of awareness of the initiative and a frequently narrow approach to policy development in schools (Smith *et al.* 1992).

Workplace health policies are also frequently narrow in focus or encounter problems of implementation; the two issues may, at least in part, be related. Cyster and McEwen (1988), for example, found that policies designed to reduce workplace problems associated with excess alcohol consumption were treated with suspicion and mistrust by employees. Embedding such policies within a wider 'healthy lifestyle' approach (along with stopping smoking, diet and exercise) made these policies more acceptable to the workforce. Further difficulties may result from a lack of guidance and training for supervisors where they are involved in implementing workplace policies on health. Cyster (1986) interviewed 70 line managers about their experiences of implementing alcohol policies and found that the majority felt they lacked adequate training and education. Even when some training does occur, this is frequently insufficient to allow programmes to be fully implemented (Cyster and McEwen 1987). With these and similar findings in mind, Christenson and Kiefhaber (1988) have argued that the more successful workplace programmes are those that are aimed at multiple risk rather than single risk behaviours, consist of environment or policy elements as well as educational interventions, are long rather than short-term or one-off programmes and are fully supported by an organizational commitment.

Creating barriers and reducing cues to unhealthy behaviour

Legislation is an efficient means of affecting the environment. The government can reduce numerous health risks by implementing laws relating to environmental pollution, public health, health and safety at work, and so on. In contrast to the potential of healthy public policy, such legislation has frequently focused on punitive measures which create barriers and reduce cues to unhealthy behaviours, most frequently in relation to tobacco and alcohol consumption. Using this approach, the promotion of healthy behaviour may be achieved through a number of processes, including taxation of unhealthy products, restricting the advertising and portrayal of unhealthy products and behaviours, and reducing the availability of unhealthy products and opportunities to engage in unhealthy behaviours. We examine evidence of the effectiveness of such measures below.

Taxation

Economic measures related to health promotion have been largely confined to taxation on tobacco and alcohol. The price of alcohol impacts on levels of consumption (e.g. Lau 1975; Central Statistics Office 1980), particularly for wines and spirits; beer consumption may be less sensitive to price (Godfrey 1990). These effects may hold not just for 'sensible' drinkers, but also those who are manifesting alcohol-related problems (Sales et al. 1989). Increases in tobacco taxation may also be the most effective measure in reducing consumption rates, with an estimated reduction in consumption of 4 per cent for every 10 per cent price rise (Peterson et al. 1992, Brownson et al. 1995).

Taxation seems to be a particularly effective deterrent among the young, who are three times more likely to be affected by price rises than older adults (Lewit et al. 1981). However, it need not be a blunt instrument. Riley (1987), for example, argued for taxation according to the alcoholic strength of drinks. This, he suggested, would increase the attractiveness of 'mid-alcohol' drinks to consumers. As a high proportion of young male drunk drivers have a blood alcohol content close to the legal limit, using legislation to encourage them to drink lower strength drinks may bring them within the legal limit without changing the number of drinks they consume.

The taxation of harmful products, particularly tobacco and alcohol, is widely supported by the public. There is less support from both consumers and producers for increasing taxation on other products such as unhealthy foods (Jeffery et al. 1990). However, fiscal policy may usefully be applied at other levels in the production process. Subsidizing farmers to grow foodstuffs instead of tobacco may, for example, support a shift from tobacco production to that of less health-damaging crops (although the European Community continued to subsidize tobacco farmers through the 1990s – in sharp contrast to the health policies of individual member countries).

Restricting advertising

Advertising may establish social norms and act as a source of social approval, reinforcing unhealthy behaviours, and possibly even mitigate against awareness of health risks. Marsh and Matheson (1983), for example, found that 44 per cent of British smokers agreed with the statement that smoking could not be really dangerous or the government would have banned cigarette advertising. Social approval may be particularly powerful when advertising is associated with sports sponsorship's image of positive health (Aitken et al. 1986).

Perhaps the most contentious advertising has been that related to tobacco and alcohol. Of particular concern has been its impact on young people. Manufacturers have argued that advertising does not encourage people to drink or smoke; rather, it serves to influence market share, encouraging those already engaged in the behaviour to purchase their product. However, advertising increases young people's awareness of cigarettes and alcohol, and shapes their attitudes relevant to these products. Under-age smokers report a preference for heavily advertised brands (Chapman and Fitzgerald 1982). Particular concern has been raised in relation to the Camel cigarette advertising campaign which began in the USA in the late 1980s. The use of the cartoon character 'Old Joe' engendered higher levels of recognition and approval among under-age smokers than adults (DiFranza et al. 1991). Similarly, Atkin et al. (1984) found that in a sample of 12 to 17-year-olds, those with higher levels of exposure to advertising were more likely to approve of under-age drinking and drunkenness.

Alexander et al. (1983) claimed that children's awareness and appreciation of advertising increased only after smoking initiation. In contrast, a number of longitudinal studies have suggested that attitudes towards cigarette advertising are predictors of future intentions and behaviour. Aitken et al. (1991), for example, interviewed a cohort of 11 to 14-year-olds in Glasgow on a number of occasions over a one-year period. Participants who expressed a strong intention to smoke when older were more aware of cigarette advertising than those who did not intend to start smoking. Those who were less responsive to cigarette advertising reported less strong intentions to smoke in the future, and these declined further over the course of the study.

Controlled studies of restricted advertising are difficult to conduct. Accordingly, evaluation of its effects has involved comparisons of consumption between countries with different advertising controls (Cox and Smith 1984), measuring the relationship between changes in advertising expenditure and consumption (Duffy 1991) and consumption levels following advertising bans (Pekurinen 1989). All of these approaches suffer from a lack of control over confounding variables. The first approach, for example, faces the problem of comparing countries that may vary greatly in terms of social attitudes, income, taxation and norms. The second approach faces problems associated with determining the direction of causality; increased advertising expenditure may be a consequence of reductions in smoking or alcohol consumption. The most reliable data is provided by a comparison of pre- and post-ban measures of consumption. The results of studies employing such a design suggest that total bans of smoking advertising are accompanied by significant falls in consumption which could not be attributed to measures such as stronger health warnings, increased education, or more rigorous enforcement of restrictions on sales to young people (Hamilton 1972; Pekurinen 1989).

Studies measuring the impact of restrictions on alcohol advertising suggest this approach may have less effect on consumption (Smart 1988). Indeed, in some cases restrictive advertising has been associated with increased consumption (Ogborne and Smart 1980). This may be due to a lack of support for such bans and a perception of alcohol consumption as socially acceptable. It seems that the 'real' price of alcohol, availability and peer behaviour appear to be more powerful determinants of consumption (Duffy 1981). Reviewing studies in this area, Maynard (1985) concluded that the association between consumption and advertising is low and that crude control of advertising 'may not be a suitable case for treatment', particularly as this may actually make alcohol cheaper.

While complete advertising bans may confer minimal advantage, control over *targeting* of such advertising may prove more necessary and effective. Young people entering the 'market' have yet to establish their regular drink, and form an attractive target group for alcohol advertising. The British alcohol industry has a code of conduct which prohibits the targeting of young people in any advertising. Nevertheless, Aitken *et al.* (1988) found that beer commercials were among the most popular commercials for children aged 13 to 14, with adverts for Carling Black Label, Miller Lite and Foster's lagers surpassing the popularity of those of Coca-Cola. Not only were these adverts popular, they were seen by this age group as conferring positive social attributes to the drinker, and served to reinforce under-age drinking. Legislation may be necessary to ensure that the industry does not target young drinkers in any future campaigns. However, the potential for satellite broadcasting to transmit programmes (and advertising) to many countries, and the European Economic Community's desire to achieve one internal market (and the difficulties of persuading some countries to adopt strict controls over advertising) may make even such controls difficult to enforce.

Restricting media portrayals

The media representation of alcohol has frequently exaggerated actual levels of consumption (DeFoe and Breed 1988/9) and focused on positive rather than negative outcomes. Drinking alcohol has been widely portrayed on the television as an acceptable social activity and personal coping strategy (Hansen 1986). In Britain, 80 per cent of popular programmes contain verbal or visual references to alcohol, with an average reference to alcohol every six minutes of programming (Smith *et al.* 1988). In the USA, analysis of prime time programmes revealed that references to alcohol doubled between 1976 and 1984, and that a majority of these references portrayed alcohol consumption in a positive light (DeFoe *et al.* 1983; Wallack *et al.* 1987). This contrasts sharply with portrayals of illicit drug use. References to this form of drug use between 1982 and 1985 occurred, on average once every four hours, with 72 per cent of references stressing negative effects (McDonald and Estep 1985). The high prevalence of positively validated uses of alcohol establishes inappropriate norms and behavioural modelling.

Restricting portrayals of unhealthy behaviours and increasing coverage of healthy behaviours in the media may influence perceptions of social norms. Van Iwaarden (1985) suggested three approaches to reducing the inappropriate portrayal of alcohol by the media: direct persuasion of opinion leaders in the electronic media, tightening up existing codes of practice on alcohol, and an information campaign targeted at all those working in the media. An even more proactive intervention has been developed by DeFoe and Breed (1988/9) in the USA, in which they drew the attention of television producers to the extent of alcohol portrayed in a number of popular programmes, provided guidelines on normalizing the portrayal of alcohol, and even offered a consulting service to develop storylines not involving alcohol.

Restricting availability

The harm consequent to tobacco consumption is a function of both the number of cigarettes smoked per day and the duration of the smoking habit. Accordingly, preventing smoking initiation or early cessation are the two most effective means of reducing smoking-related harm. One way of facilitating this approach is to prevent young people's access to tobacco and tobacco products. While such legislation exists in many countries, there have been many problems in preventing the sale of tobacco to minors. The issue for health promotion to address here may not be the establishment of appropriate legislation, but its enforcement (Cummings *et al.* 1994). With this in mind, Brownson *et al.* (1995) have called for a licence system for tobacco sales, which could be revoked if laws are broken, similar to that used to control alcohol sales.

Despite such a licensing system restrictions on the sale of alcohol to minors has encountered similar problems to those related to tobacco. However, a report by Jeffs and Saunders (1983) provides one example of how these problems may be overcome through modest changes in police practice. They established high-profile community policing during the tourist season at an English seaside resort. On a regular basis over the summer period, two or three uniformed policemen entered the local bars and public houses and amicably checked for under-age drinking and the unsociable drunk. This simple strategy resulted in a substantial reduction in crime (and particularly that which was alcohol-related) in the intervention area, when compared with projected figures and those of a control town.

Whether the early consumption of alcohol leads to later drink-related problems is a moot point. However, the short-term consequences of inebriation may differ according to age. Accordingly, there has been substantial interest in studies exploring the impact of changing the age of legal drinking on short-term negative consequences of consumption. Perhaps the most important of these is a series of studies evaluating the effect of differing ages of legal consumption on rates of road traffic accidents involving drink-driving. Such comparisons have been possible as a consequence of US state drinking laws which may differ between states and over time. Unfortunately, no clear effect has emerged. Some studies have identified little or no effect of such legislation (e.g. Hingson *et al.* 1983; Choukron *et al.* 1985), while others have suggested that increasing the age of legal consumption reduces the prevalence of drink-related accidents. Wagenaar (1983), for example, compared data from Maine and Michigan, which first reduced then raised the legal age of drinking. Although the magnitude of the impact of legislation differed between the two states, a clear reduction in accidents involving both injury and damage to property was found following increases in the drinking age from 18 to 20 years. The Fatal Accident Reporting System (National Highway Traffic Safety Administration 1988) also reported a 30 per cent fall in fatal traffic accidents involving drink-drivers in states that raised their legal drinking age from 16 to 21 years between 1982 and 1986. States that did not change the minimum age to 21 also showed a reduction, but only by 19 per cent. More conservatively, Asch and Levy (1987) suggested that it is the experience of alcohol rather than the age at which consumption begins which is the intervening variable. Their results suggested that regardless of age, those in their first year of drinking had a 10 to 20 per cent higher fatality risk than the rest of the driving population.

Drink-driving legislation has typically been enforced through the identification and apprehension of obviously drunk drivers. However, despite some negative findings (Mercer 1985; Ross *et al.* 1987) there is increasing evidence that well publicized roadside checks, particularly those incorporating educational programmes, can significantly reduce both crash and fatality rates (Eperlein 1985). A complementary or alternative legislative approach is to ensure appropriate punishment for those found guilty of alcohol-related driving offences. An example of such an approach is that adopted by Sweden, where offenders with a blood alcohol count greater than 150 mg per 100 ml receive imprisonment for up to one year or 25 'day-fines' (25/ 1000 of annual income). If their blood alcohol count is within the range of 50–150 mg, they receive a fine of 10 'day-fines'. Both groups receive automatic licence withdrawal. The value of such an approach lies in its equity, although its effectiveness in comparison with other legislative procedures may be more difficult to ascertain.

Restriction of the availability of previously available unhealthy products is a controversial and politically sensitive measure. Its effectiveness is also unclear. Severe restrictions of the availability of alcohol in Poland, Sweden and a number of other countries resulted in substantial reductions in official consumption figures (although the use of illegal stills and distribution networks suggests that these effects are probably exaggerated). However, less stringent approaches to the reduction of availability in Australia, Canada and some states of the USA have resulted in no changes in consumption (Schnelle et al. 1975; Smart and Docherty 1976). In addition, the political acceptability of such an approach is negligible and this approach cannot be considered a viable option.

More modest restrictions in access may be more acceptable. Godfrey (1990) suggested two mechanisms by which limiting the number of retail outlets may reduce demand for alcohol. First, restricted numbers of outlets may increase transaction costs (travel, time, and so on). Second, the outlets themselves (and posters and logos near them) act as advertising; restricting outlets would therefore restrict advertising. Evidence in support of such a notion comes from a study by Holder (1987) who made use of the fact that in 1978 some counties in North Carolina changed their laws on the sale of liquor in licensed clubs and restaurants. Before the change, patrons could bring their own bottle of liquor and purchase ice and glasses. After the change they could purchase liquor by the glass at the place of consumption. Comparisons between those counties which implemented these changes and those that did not revealed a 250 per cent increase in establishments where liquor could be purchased. This was associated with an increase in sales of distilled spirits ranging from 6 to 7.4 per cent and an increase in traffic accidents of between 16 and 24 per cent.

Evidence on the dangers of passive smoking has formed a catalyst for restrictive smoking policies (NRC 1986). Nearly two-thirds of US worksites with a workforce of more than 50 people are thought to have a smoking restriction policy (USDHHS 1993). In Britain, *The Health of the Nation* (Department of Health 1992) strategy document stated that 80 per cent of public places, such as cinemas and shops, should have established a no smoking policy by 1994. Workplace policies that have restrictive smoking policies combined with education or cessation programmes have proven the most effective methods of reducing smoking prevalence within the workforce (Fielding 1982, see also Chapter 7). Similarly, in schools the presence of a no smoking policy combined with health education appears to be the most effective way of minimizing tobacco consumption among pupils (Pentz et al. 1989). However, behavioural norms may vary according to setting. Moore (1996) noted that British bars and public houses remain one of the few settings in which cigarette smoking remains the norm. Here, restrictions, rather than total bans, are supported by the majority of patrons. Similar findings have been reported in Australia (Schofield and Edwards 1995), where only 20 per cent of drinkers supported a total ban on smoking in bars, while 65 per cent supported the establishment of smoking areas.

Changing the social environment

Health promotion programmes can be used to change social norms and to teach skills of resistance to the influence of unhealthy norms. Perceived social norms may be changed through educative processes or modelling appropriate healthy norms. Skills provision may involve training in assertiveness or refusal skills. The majority of such interventions have taken place within schools, and combined these various processes with the use of peer educators (Schaps et al. 1981). The last element has a number of advantages (Klepp et al. 1986). Peers may influence informational norms through modelling healthy behaviours. They may also foster the development of assertion and resistance skills through vicarious learning from role play and behavioural modelling. Peers may also possess more credibility as sources of information than teachers, particularly in discussion of the use of illicit drugs (Perry et al. 1986).

Peers are not the only influence on young people's perceptions of, and resistance to, social norms. Amos (1992) suggested that the influence of parents' smoking behaviour on their children requires their involvement in school educational programmes. Interestingly, this involvement may have a reciprocal effect on parental behaviour. Charlton (1988), for example, found that such programmes not only reduced the uptake of smoking by the children, they also reduced parental smoking levels. However the effectiveness of using parents to change children's perceptions of social norms is unclear (Green and Iverson 1982). Overall, it seems effective for younger children but for older children it may be counterproductive. Here, there may be a rejection of the perceived behavioural norms of adults. In addition, the needs of this age group may be to focus on independent decision-making skills.

There is increasing evidence that peer-led interventions may be effective, and more so than conventional teaching approaches, in the context of substance abuse programmes. Schaps et al. (1981) reviewed the effectiveness of 127 schools-based drug abuse prevention programmes involving 10 types of teaching methods. Over half involved the didactic teaching of relevant facts. One-third focused on attempts to persuade pupils not to abuse drugs, while a quarter involved the teaching of assertion and decision-making skills.

A smaller percentage focused on strengthening or exploiting peer dynamics which inhibited drugs use, and family strategies. Teachers were the predominant leaders of this teaching, with peers leading 5 per cent of programmes and parents leading only 1 per cent.

The outcome of each programme was rated on a scale from +3 indicating a substantially positive effect to a −3 for a substantially negative effect. The most effective were those which focused on family strategies for avoiding drug usage (overall rating = +0.79). Peer strategies and skills building achieved a similar level of success (rating +0.55). Persuasion and didactic information provision were the least successful methods (with scores of +0.45 and +0.29 respectively). When mode of delivery was examined, the average outcome rating for peer-led programmes was +1.25, for parent-led programmes +1.0, and for teachers +0.40. These differences, while indicative, did not achieve statistical significance as the programme categories were not mutually exclusive and there were a small number of peer-led and skills-based programmes. However, the authors argue that the results reflect findings in individual studies.

In one such study, Bachman et al. (1988) evaluated a programme in which students were encouraged to talk about drugs to each other, to state their disapproval of drug usage, and to assert that they did not take drugs. This encouraged an informational social norm that was anti-drug taking and fostered verbal refusal skills. This intervention resulted in changed attitudes towards drugs and drug use, and a decrease in marijuana use. Sussman et al. (1995) examined three different approaches to substance misuse prevention in a Californian study involving nearly 1000 young people. Pupils were selected from 12 schools and allocated to either a traditional information lesson on drug use, a lesson focusing on resisting social norm pressure, or a programme designed to correct erroneous informational social influence. Half the pupils received a teacher-led programme, while the other intervention required active pupil participation. Significant changes in attitudes and intentions not to use drugs were reported in the programmes involving active participation, but not the teacher-led programmes.

Less research has been conducted to evaluate the impact of peer-led and social norm-based initiatives in relation to other health areas. However, there is some evidence that they may be equally effective in HIV education. Klepp et al. (1994) reported a study conducted in Africa, in which they evaluated a two to three-month long school education programme designed to increase knowledge of HIV transmission, discussion of safer sex practices, and tolerance for people with AIDS (PWAs). It was also designed to reduce the incidence of 'risky sex'. The programme attempted to encourage a social norm that supported celibacy and, as a consequence, reduced intentions to engage in sexual intercourse. Classes received an average of 20 hours of education using a wide variety of techniques from teachers who had received specific training and a teachers' manual. Following the intervention, those pupils who were involved in the programme reported higher levels of exposure to information communication about AIDS and knowledge than those of a control group. They also had more positive attitudes towards PWAs, a more restrictive subjective norm and reported less intentions to engage in sexual intercourse.

Social normative influence may also play a role in the promotion of health among adults. The majority of programmes drawing on such an approach have been confined to the workplace. This setting provides a context in which it is possible to reach the largest number of people and their dependants, for most years of their adult life (Pelletier 1993). It also provides the opportunity for social support and the opportunity to participate with friends and co-workers. A study reported by Zimmerman and Connor (1989) illustrates the importance of social support in facilitating behavioural change at the worksite. They examined the moderating influence of naturally occurring differences in social support on the outcome of a workplace health promotion programme. The programme involved attendance at seven group sessions, each lasting one and a half hours, focusing on the following: controlling health, risk appraisal, physical fitness, nutrition, stress management, goal setting and feedback. Pre-intervention measures were taken on a range of health behaviours, including smoking, salt use, diet and exercise, as well as expectations of support from family friends and co-workers. Immediately following the intervention, the behavioural measures were repeated. In addition, participants rated how important support from family, friends and co-workers had been in facilitating and maintaining behavioural change.

Prior to the intervention, the majority of participants expected all three groups to be supportive of change; 89 per cent expected their family to support them, and 75 per cent expected the friends and co-workers to support them. These expectations were moderately optimistic. Following the intervention, 75 per cent stated their family had been supportive, while two-thirds considered their friends and co-workers to have given them some support. Support from at least one source contributed significantly to changes in dietary fat intake, increases in exercise, and a measure of overall risk behaviour reduction. The influence of such social support, additional to any programme effects, suggests that it could usefully be incorporated more formally within health promotion initiatives. Involving co-workers and families in programmes could facilitate behavioural change via mutually supportive social support.

Unfortunately, many of the interventions carried out in the worksite have failed to take advantage of the potential of the social environment to foster or maintain change. However, Erfurt et al. (1990) provided one example of how social norms may be utilized to facilitate participation in health promotion programmes within the workplace. They compared participation rates in three contrasting interventions provided at different worksites: health screening alone, screening in combination with health education classes, and a more complex intervention. This involved screening and health education classes combined with changes to the social and physical environment, including the setting up of buddy systems, health competitions, increasing exercise facilities and encouraging increased exercise at the plant. Participation rates in the two major programmes of weight loss and smoking cessation were 46 and 54 per cent respectively in the latter programme. These compared with participation rates of less than 10 per cent in the site offering only health education classes and of less than 1 per cent in the screening-only site.

Another study in the workplace (Brownell and Felix 1987) utilized social norms to increase participation and adherence to a weight reduction programme. Participants were organized into competitive teams, given relevant self-help manuals and a baseline weight assessment was conducted. Throughout the programme, the results from weekly weigh-ins were displayed in a prominent position at each worksite. This was intended to change perceptions of social norms and increase social support as well as provide feedback on how each team was progressing in comparison with its competitors. After approximately 15 weeks, attrition was less than 1 per cent and average weight loss was 5.5 kg. This degree of weight loss is impressive, and the authors considered the intervention to be a success. However, the long-term consequences of establishing competitive in- and out-groups can often be less constructive (Sherif and Hovland 1961) and this form of intervention needs to be conducted with care.

Summary and conclusions

We have identified a number of theories and psychological processes which may provide a theoretical underpinning to many structuralist approaches. Some environmental manipulations will clearly affect health regardless of their behavioural consequences. Improvements in housing quality and medical services may impact on health directly and without behavioural mediation. However, a number of environmental manipulations are effective because of their impact on behaviour. Two sets of environmental interventions appear important: those which increase the likelihood of individuals engaging in health-enhancing behaviours; and those which reduce the likelihood of health-damaging behaviours. The former include providing cues to healthy behaviour, appropriate product labelling and environmental changes at both the local and national level. The latter involves restrictive legislation and taxation. A further change of the social environment involves changing social norms to be more supportive of health-protective behaviours.

Public health policy is potentially an extremely powerful means of facilitating behavioural change and public health. However, it involves not only health but the political process. The decision of the British government not to ban the advertising of cigarettes, for example, has not been based on the evidence of the impact of such legislation on health. Rather, it was the result of a political process, with other agendas and priorities. Future health promotion priorities need not only to formulate effective environmental policies, but to develop strategies to facilitate their implementation. Such policies may need to focus on positive incentives rather than punitive approaches and integrate skills-based or norm-based interventions with wider environmental changes.

Suggested reading

Bunton, R., Nettleton, S. and Burrows, R. (1995) *The Sociology of Health Promotion*. London: Routledge.

Davies, J. and Kelly, M. (eds) (1993) *Healthy Cities: Research and Practice*. London: Routledge.

Glanz, K., Lankenau, B., Foerster, S., Temple, S., Mullis, R. and Schmid, T. (1995) Environmental and policy approaches to cardiovascular disease prevention through nutrition: opportunities for state and local action. *Health Education Quarterly*, 22: 512–27.

Hancock, T. (1993) The evolution, impact and significance of the healthy cities/healthy communities movement. *Journal of Public Health Policy*, 14: 5–18.

Tonnes, K. and Tilford, S. (1994) *Health Education: Effectiveness, Efficiency and Equity*. (2nd edn). London: Chapman and Hall.

CHAPTER
6

Attitude and communication theories

Health promotion has implicitly and explicitly drawn on a number of communication and attitude theories to inform mass media campaigns and the
use of media resources such as videos, leaflets and posters. Research in this
area can be broadly divided into two areas: 'laboratory' studies (which
include school and clinic-based evaluations), and evaluations of mass media
campaigns and communication processes within the community.

The first method offers the opportunity not only to control the intervention but to manipulate elements such as source and message content within
it. Such studies frequently lack external validity, as responses to media campaigns in the real world are rarely so controlled. However, what evaluations
of community campaigns gain in external validity, they lose in terms of
control over potentially confounding variables. Media output is frequently
combined with other interventions, making it impossible to specify the effects
of media interventions alone (Puska *et al.* 1985). Evaluations typically compare differences between people who report having seen the media output
and those who do not. This may result in inappropriate comparisons;
memory biases, for example, may result in allocation to the wrong group. In
addition, most studies report cross-sectional designs in which comparisons
are made between measures taken after the media programme. This makes
it difficult to establish the media output per se as having contributed to these
differences, as there may be pre-existing differences between these groups.
Viewers and non-viewers of television health campaigns frequently differ
on measures of information-seeking behaviour, health knowledge and educational status, as well as the frequency in which they engage in the behaviour
in question (Lau *et al.* 1980; Bennett *et al.* 1991b).

For these reasons, the focus of research conducted within the laboratory
or community has differed markedly. Laboratory studies have primarily
focused on fine-grain analysis of the characteristics of media output and its
recipients that moderate its effectiveness in changing attitudes and behaviour.

Those in community settings have focused on how messages initially transmitted through the media are understood and diffused through the wider community. We adopt this dichotomy in the present chapter, focusing initially on laboratory studies before examining research conducted in the community.

Laboratory-based research

Laboratory-based research has concentrated on measuring the effect of varying sources of information, message content, and recipient characteristics on knowledge, attitude and behavioural intention. One particular message variable, that of threat or fear arousal, has been of particular interest to many communication researchers. Social learning theory (Bandura 1977) and the health belief model (Becker 1974) can be seen as implicitly informing such an approach. Social learning theory suggests that fear messages act as a threat of punishment, often in the long term, if a course of action is not adopted. Similarly, the health belief model suggests that fear involves perceived vulnerability to threat and the perceived severity of that threat. Two further theories have been used to examine the use of fear messages within health promotion: the dual process model (Leventhal et al. 1983) and protection motivation theory (Maddux and Rogers 1983). A third theory which we outline, the elaboration likelihood model (Petty and Cacioppo 1986), focuses more on the match between message and recipient characteristics.

The dual process model

The dual process model posits a bilateral response to health-threatening communication. Leventhal and colleagues (1983) suggest that fear messages lead to two parallel sets of cognitive processing. The first, danger control, involves evaluation of the threat and how to deal with it. The second, fear control, involves consideration of how to cope with any emotional reaction to this threat. Fear control acts as a motivating force towards the adoption of attitudes supporting threat-reducing behavioural change (danger control). The emotional reaction may be short-lived, but the cognitive representation of the danger and a coping plan remain in longer-term memory. However, fear messages may lead to such strong emotional reactions that valid cognitive representations of the health threat are prevented from forming. In such cases no coping plan or preventive behaviour would result.

Protection motivation theory

Protection motivation theory combines elements of social learning theory and the health belief model to provide a model of how fear-arousing health communications are processed and acted upon. The model focuses on two broad categories of response: threat appraisal and coping appraisal. The outcome of this appraisal process is an intention to behave in either an adaptive or maladaptive manner (Boer and Seydel 1996), the strength of which reflects the degree of motivation to protect one's health. This intention, in turn, predicts behaviour.

As in the health belief model, threat appraisal is a function of both the perceived susceptibility to illness and its severity. Consideration is also given to the benefits of maintaining maladaptive behaviours. Coping appraisal is a function of both outcome and self-efficacy beliefs. Accordingly, an individual is most likely to change their behaviour in response to a fear-arousing health message if they believe they are susceptible to disease, that the disease will have severe consequences, they perceive a link between protective behaviours and reduced risk for disease, and consider themselves capable of engaging in them.

Although similar to the health belief model, there are some important differences between the two theories. First, the health belief model is a general theory of health-behaviour decision-making; protection motivation theory is a model of responses to fear-arousing communications. Second, the notion of self-efficacy is more explicitly defined in protection motivation theory. Although self-efficacy judgements may be relevant to an evaluation of costs involved in engaging in health-promoting behaviour, the process of both outcome expectancies and self-efficacy are more explicit and circumscribed. Third, health motivation is a derived and guiding intention in protection motivation theory. In the health belief model it is less well-defined, and does not have such a central role; it is merely one of several factors seen to influence behaviour.

The elaboration likelihood model

The elaboration likelihood model suggests that the influence of media output is the result of an interaction between message factors and the cognitive state of the recipient. It states that individuals are differentially motivated to attend to and process media messages as a consequence of their pre-existing beliefs and interests. They are more likely to attend to messages if they are 'motivated to receive an argument', because it is congruent with their pre-existing beliefs, has personal relevance to them, or they have the intellectual capacity to consider and process any message (Sherif and Hovland 1961; Apsler and Sears 1968). Where these conditions exist, individuals engage in what Petty and Cacioppo refer to as central processing. This involves evaluation of arguments, assessment of conclusions, and their integration within existing belief structures. Any attitudinal change consequent to such processing is likely to be enduring over time. Media messages attempting to facilitate such a process should focus on strong arguments rather than style, be clear and understandable and reflect recipients' existing beliefs (Sorrentino et al. 1988).

In contrast, recipients who are unmotivated to receive an argument, who have low issue involvement or incongruent beliefs are more likely to respond to the credibility and attractiveness of the source. Identified as peripheral processing, any resultant attitudinal change is likely to be transient and not predictive of behaviour. This group may also be more responsive to emotional message appeals.

Communication and recipient characteristics as moderators of impact

Rather than review the literature in a piecemeal manner, focusing on each theory in turn, we assess the importance of aspects of each theory within a more traditional framework of communication research, addressing the impact of source, message and receiver characteristics on the impact of any media output. We identify issues relevant to each theory as we progress.

Source characteristics

Research from the 1950s and beyond has consistently shown that the characteristics of those providing information through the media impact on its effectiveness (e.g. Petty and Cacioppo 1986; Wu and Shaffer 1987). These may vary on a number of dimensions, including attractiveness, credibility, perceived power, and similarity to the target audience. The importance of the source may increase when comprehension of message content or the strength of argument is low (Ratneshwar and Chaiken 1991), although even where the strength of argument is considered high, source characteristics retain some influence on message impact (DeBono and Telesca 1990). Indeed, even when a message is initially rejected due to its source characteristics it can become persuasive over time (Gruder et al. 1978). This can occur if the message content has a high impact, when information about the source is received after its content, or as a consequence of the message becoming disassociated from its source over time (Kelman and Hovland 1953).

Sources that are liked and considered similar to the receiver are more likely to be considered attractive and to improve recall and attitude change than disliked or dissimilar sources (DeBono and Telesca 1990). As predicted by the elaboration likelihood model, the attractiveness of the source is most important where comprehension of message content is low (Ratneshwar and Chaiken 1991). One explanation for this influence may be found in cognitive dissonance theory (Festinger 1957). This suggests that that attractiveness may act as a form of external justification for attitude change, allowing us to restore cognitive consonance when we are asked to do something we are opposed to. Popular sources (such as famous sports personalities or comedians) and those matched to recipients by demographic variables could therefore play an important part in changing resistant attitudes and behaviour.

Source credibility refers both to expertise and trustworthiness. The latter appears to be particularly important. Sources that are disinterested in outcomes, or who state an interest in outcomes before a message is seen, are considered more trustworthy than sources who are considered likely to gain from any attitudinal or behavioural change (McGuire 1985). For this reason, experts from government and the medical establishment may be considered less trustworthy than lay experts, such as ex- or current drug users. Direct exposure to such an attitude object is likely to result in attitudinal change which is more resistant to counter-arguments and predictive of behaviour than those engendered by more neutral sources or information mediated through sources such as television (Fazio and Zanna 1981; Wu and Shaffer 1987).

Emotional involvement with the source of any message may also increase its impact (e.g. Solomon and DeJong 1986). However, where such processes are utilized they may form only part of a powerful interplay between positive emotional involvement and stereotypes, prejudice and stigma. A number of examples of these subtle processes may be found in media messages related to HIV and AIDS. Scollay *et al.* (1992) reported that a message source known to be HIV positive or have AIDS resulted in greater increases in knowledge, less risky attitudes, and safer behavioural intentions than a neutral source. More subtle effects were reported by Dennehey *et al.* (1995). They evaluated the effect of an AIDS prevention lecture given by a confederate who posed as an HIV positive person who had become infected through one of four routes: heterosexual transmission, homosexual transmission, blood transfusion, or sharing needles. The content of each 20-minute lecture was the same, covering transmission, prevention and treatment of AIDS. Control groups either received a lecture from a neutral presenter or had no lecture.

As expected, knowledge scores increased in all the AIDS lecture conditions in comparison to the control conditions. However, knowledge scores increased most in the heterosexual and transfusion conditions. Overall, the HIV positive lecturer was rated more trustworthy, expert and attractive than the neutral lecturer. However, the lecturer in the heterosexual condition was seen as more expert than in the drug using condition and more trustworthy than in the homosexual and drug using condition. Here, attributions of blame and responsibility appear to have influenced subjects' responses to differing communication sources.

Message content

Many variables can affect the impact of media message, including: one versus two-sided arguments, the provision of conclusions, forcefulness, rational versus emotional content and levels of fear. We briefly summarize data from a number of studies which have examined the impact of such variables, before focusing on studies evaluating the effect of emotional messages, particularly fear arousal.

As predicted by the elaboration likelihood model, messages which provide arguments from two sides of an issue are more effective than didactic one-sided messages with individuals who are at the stage of contemplating behaviour change (Hovland *et al.* 1949), have higher levels of education (McGuire 1985) or who know that the issue is complex or controversial (Baumgardner *et al.* 1983). When the issue being addressed is a complex one or audiences are easily distracted, messages that contain a conclusion or recommendations are more effective than those that do not. In contrast, when the issue is relatively straightforward, allowing audiences to draw their own conclusions is frequently most effective (Linder and Worchel 1970). Messages delivered in a more forceful style are particularly persuasive and may be harder for audiences to counter-argue. Forcefulness can be enhanced by such things as pitch variation, extreme descriptions, the use of specific examples and higher volume (Robinson and McArthur 1982).

A number of social cognition and communication models identify threat, or more starkly fear, as a factor motivating attitudinal or behavioural change. The emphasis they place on threat varies considerably. The health belief model and protection motivation theory place threat perception as a central process of behavioural mediation; the health action process (Schwarzer 1992) considers threat to be much more peripheral. However, no model considers threat to be the only factor involved. In contrast, many media campaigns have considered threat, or fear arousal, as the primary determinant of behaviour.

Early studies of the impact of fear-arousing communications simply manipulated levels of fear. A study by Janis and Feshbach (1953) exemplifies this type of study. It involved three conditions in which high school students sat through a 15-minute lecture and slide presentation on dental hygiene. Level of threat was manipulated by varying the degree of personally threatening slides in each presentation. Immediately after the presentations, students in the high arousal group reported higher levels of motivation to care for their teeth than the other groups. One week later, however, they had retained less information and their behaviour did not differ from that of any other group. Similar results have been found in relation to smoking cessation (Janis and Terwilliger 1962), motivation to buy condoms (Rhodes and Wolitski 1990) and in alcohol misuse (Smart and Fejer 1974; Fritzen and Mazer 1975).

Rather than motivate behavioural change, moderate or high fear may actually interfere with change (Leventhal *et al.* 1983). Fear-arousing messages have encouraged resistance to the message (Franzkowiak 1987), increased denial that a threat applies to the individual (Soames-Job 1988) and even increased the behaviour they were attempting to counter. Following fear-based campaigns, the prevalence of both illicit drug usage (Louira 1988), and drink-driving (Malfetti 1985) have risen. Even where significant and persistent health concerns are raised, behaviour change may not follow. The Australian AIDS initiative conducted in the 1980s known as the 'Grim Reaper campaign' increased audience awareness of AIDS and measures of health anxiety. However, it had no impact on knowledge or sexual behaviour (Rigby *et al.* 1989).

Fear messages may not always be counter-productive. They may motivate change under conditions of low levels of perceived vulnerability (Watts 1968; Higbee 1969), high self-esteem (Rosen *et al.* 1982) and high self-efficacy (Maddux and Rogers 1983; Stretcher *et al.* 1986). In general, however, they have resulted in minimal change. They also have potential disadvantages. Within HIV education, for example, high fear content messages have encouraged an increase in coercive attitudes towards people with AIDS (Allard 1989). Despite these consistent findings, audiences frequently consider high-fear messages to be more effective than low-fear messages in influencing behaviour (Rhodes and Wolitski 1990), perhaps explaining their popularity among government funding agencies and politicians.

Threat or fear may be conveyed in a number of subtle ways. For example, health messages can be framed in either positive or negative terms. Negative frames may make messages more memorable than positive ones (Newhagen and Reeves 1987). Meyerowitz and Chaiken (1987) examined the effect of positively and negatively framed messages on women's breast self-examination. Their positive messages stressed the health benefits while the negative messages concentrated on the potential dangers of failing to self-examine. The negative messages had a greater influence on the women's attitudes to examination, intentions and behaviour when measured four months later. Conversely, Isen (1987) suggested that a positive rather than a negative mood results in individuals processing information more quickly, with less effort and less thought. Individuals in a positive mood may also reach conclusions based on less information and may be more likely to stick to them. Mackie *et al.* (1990) found that positive moods were associated with more attention being paid to the credibility of the source and less to the quality of the message. Positive messages may therefore be more effective than negative messages when elaboration time is minimal and peripheral processing occurs, with the reverse the case when elaboration is maximized (Maheswaran and Meyers-Levy 1990). Flora and Maibach (1990) suggested that both negative and positive emotional messages are more memorable when individuals can compare them to a message with the opposite emotional valence. It may be the contrast that is important, not the effect.

So far we have considered the impact of messages with a high fear or threat component without regard to other components of the communication. It is possible that threat messages in combination with other elements may be more effective in facilitating change. Both Solomon and DeJong (1986) and Kenny (1989) suggest that fear messages will be effective when means of avoiding the feared outcome are also provided. Behavioural alternatives need to be offered which individuals feel are manageable and effective and will lead to a reduction in threat (Meichenbaum 1974; Perloff 1993). These arguments reflect the central tenets of protection motivation theory and social learning theory.

A number of studies have compared the predictive strength of fear arousal with other potentially important cognitive variables. Plotnikoff and Higginbotham (1995), for example, examined the relationship between intentions to lower dietary fat intake and threat appraisal, outcome expectations, and self-efficacy measures in a general population sample in Australia. They found no relationship between threat appraisal and intentions to eat a low fat diet. However, outcome expectations and self-efficacy judgements were significantly associated with intentions to change diet. The low correlation between threat appraisal and behavioural intentions and behaviour has been replicated on a number of occasions (Schwarzer 1992). However, some evidence of the importance of threat as a behavioural motivator has been found.

In a direct test of protection motivation theory, Boer and Seydel (1996) measured the impact of a leaflet accompanying an invitation to attend a mass screening clinic for breast cancer. The leaflet described the high vulnerability of older women to breast cancer and the high response efficacy of mammographic screening as a means of cancer control. It also attempted to induce feelings of high self-efficacy by explaining that a mammographic examination was an easy procedure and involved only minimal discomfort. Women who rated themselves as most vulnerable to breast cancer and who had high self-efficacy were most likely to intend to attend screening. Similarly, Bennett and Rowe (in press) found a significant correlation between the perceived threat of an episode of asthma and adherence to a preventive medication regime. Neither outcome expectancies nor efficacy beliefs were predictive.

Recipient characteristics

The elaboration likelihood model suggests that people with low issue involvement are more responsive to emotional appeals than reasoned argument. Accordingly, Flora and Maibach (1990) have argued that the role of emotion in health education may be as a motivator of those unaware of risks. Models of coping have provided further understanding of how individuals may react to media messages. Byrne (1961) identified two broad coping styles. The first, similar to Lazarus and Folkman's (1984) construct of problem focused coping, he termed monitoring or sensitization. The second, analogous to emotion focused coping, he called blunting or repression. Individuals with a monitoring style tend to seek out information about health threats while those with a blunting style ignore or distract themselves from it. Previous exposure to health promotion initiatives or relevant health information may also influence responses. McGuire (1964) identified a process of inoculation which occurs when individuals are exposed to arguments against existing attitudes or behaviours. Exposure to weak arguments can provide the individual with an opportunity to rehearse counter-arguments and may increase their resistance to subsequent messages even if these are intrinsically persuasive.

Prevailing cultural and social norms may also moderate the influence of any media output (Ajzen and Fishbein 1980). Messages may be more influential if they are from an in-group rather than out-group source (Wilder 1990). However, two similar studies by the same research team suggest the variability of this effect, at least on issues not specific to particular groups. In the first (Ramirez and Lasater 1977), ethnic similarity between communicator and recipient produced greater compliance following dental health education than ethnic dissimilarity. This result was not replicated in their second study (Dembroski et al. 1978). A similar picture emerges when gender is considered. Some studies suggest that men respond more than women to both high and low fear content messages (Struckman-Johnson et al. 1990) and that age is negatively correlated with the effectiveness of a fear approach (Rhodes and Wolitski 1990). In contrast, Carter and Carter (1993) found that females were more responsive to all messages regardless of content, while Sawyer and Beck (1991) found no gender differences in susceptibility to either affective and rational appeals. Such disparate findings highlight the need for well-designed evaluation studies that examine how the interaction of factors such as age, gender and ethnicity affect responses to interventions. These relationships are likely to be subtle. Carli (1990), for example, found that a female who spoke tentatively on an issue was more persuasive than one who spoke assertively with a male audience, while the reverse was true for female audiences. Interestingly there were no gender differences when a male source was used.

Communication through communities

The impact of media output in real life differs significantly from that within the laboratory. Its messages may be less well attended to, and may be accepted or rejected as a consequence of social attitudes and social norms. In turn, they may influence these norms, and attitudinal or behavioural change may occur not as a consequence of direct exposure to a media programme, but indirectly as a consequence of other people's attitude or behaviour change. Health promotion initiatives are also subject to competition from other sources within the social environment. These include other media outputs; advertising for cigarettes and alcohol, for example, may compete with health promotion messages directly. More subtly, the models of behaviour provided through media programming may influence attitudes and behaviour. These various issues have led to theories attempting to explain the process of communication within social systems. We introduce two of the most commonly cited in health promotion here: diffusion of innovation theory (Rogers 1983) and social marketing (Lefebvre and Flora 1988).

Diffusion of innovation

The process of diffusion of innovation (Rogers, 1983) attempts to explain the spread of new ideas and behaviours within society. Like other communication theories (McGuire 1985), it recognizes that individuals progress through a number of stages if behaviour change is to occur: initial awareness and increased knowledge of an innovation; persuasion, where attitudes to favourable adoption occur; a decision to test out the innovation on a trial basis; and then adoption. However diffusion theory also recognizes that the mass media is only one channel of potential influence, competing with other channels of information and being interpreted and reinterpreted through social networks. Three main variables are posited to explain this process. They emphasize the importance of the characteristics of the innovation, the classification of individuals within communities, and the importance of interpersonal communication.

For an innovation to be successfully diffused it needs to possess a number of characteristics. It should involve minimal costs or commitment, be simple to understand or implement and should result in observable benefits. In this, the theory shares assumptions with social learning theory, the health belief model and protection motivation theory (see Chapter 2). In addition the innovation needs to be perceived as part of the social norm: that is, consistent with the existing values and experiences of the audience. Here, the theory is consonant with the theories of reasoned action and planned behaviour (Ajzen and Fishbein 1980; Ajzen 1985).

Typically the entry and legitimization of an innovation follows an S-shaped trajectory; slow initial uptake is followed by a rapid acceptance and a final slowing as a minority, termed laggards, resist acceptance. Early acceptors, typically those from a high socio-economic group and atypical of the community they live within are classed as innovators. They are often information seekers and account for a very small percentage of those adopting an innovation in a population. However, their behaviour brings the innovation to the attention of opinion leaders within the community who are more typical, have good communication networks and status. These early adopters make the innovation visible and communicate its benefits to others. Once their attention is drawn to the innovation, the next group, the early majority decide whether or not to adopt the innovation following a deliberative assessment of costs and benefits. The fourth group, known as the late majority, typically have lower social status, are more sceptical and gain information from those around them, rather than other sources. Accordingly, behaviour change is likely to be the result of conformity to social norms rather than an assessment of costs and benefits. Finally, the laggards tend to be socially isolated and traditional in behaviour; they are thought to change through compliance to the majority.

Two different modes of transmission of innovations through society can be identified. Mediated channels such as television and newspapers retain a distance in time and space between source and receiver; non-mediated channels such as health professionals, teachers, families and peers provide a direct link. Mediated channels may be most effective in gaining attention and arousing interest and non-mediated channels more effective in delivering intense persuasive messages and complex information (Bettinghaus 1986). Accordingly, the mass media may play an important role during early diffusion, raising awareness and communicating basic information, and influencing early adopters in particular. Non-mediated channels become important at later stages as a consequence of their ability to provide informational social influence, and may prove particularly effective in influencing late adopters.

Diffusion of innovations involves change agencies who develop innovations, change agents who communicate information about and promote the innovation, and recipients of the innovation. Havelock (1974) suggested that rapid diffusion is more likely to occur if the decision is imposed from above by relatively few in a social system, such as a change agency, rather than from below and collectively. However, it is important to note that change can occur within social groups without any outside change agency. A recognition of problems, the need for change, and potential solutions can occur spontaneously within communities and a similar process of diffusion can occur. This can be seen in the increase of media advocacy to promote policy initiatives and counteract unhealthy media messages, and the rise of health coalition groups such as ASH (Action for Smoking and Health) and the Terrence Higgins Trust which provide a political and economic voice to those particularly interested in increasing awareness and political action on specific health issues.

Measuring the spread of innovations, and formal testing of diffusion of innovation theory, is a difficult process. As the diffusion process can be spread over a long period of time, appropriate evaluation requires longitudinal studies and detailed process research, conducted at key points in the hypothesized S-distribution. The costs involved in conducting such research have meant that the majority of studies have depended on respondent recall of environmental and behavioural changes within cross-sectional designs with little objective verification of self-reports (Macdonald 1992). Accordingly, while diffusion of innovation theory has high face validity, its empirical status has yet to be fully understood.

Social marketing

The importance placed on understanding audience characteristics when designing media campaigns and the use of targeted, rather than mass campaigns, has led to the increased use of social marketing techniques. These apply the principles of commercial marketing to health promotion, through exchange theory and a consumer orientation. Such an approach involves audience segmentation, formative research and channel analysis and results in a particular marketing mix for the 'product'. It is not without its critics who have argued against the dangers of treating health as a commodity much as other commodities in the marketplace (Nettleton and Bunton 1995). However, it may prove a valuable means of identifying target groups within larger populations and help to identify the form of intervention most appropriate to each group (e.g. Black and Smith 1994; Cirksena and Flora 1995).

Slater and Flora (1991) afford an example of the use of audience segmentation to determine relevant health promotion approaches using survey data from the Stanford Five Cities project. They identified clusters of individuals within the city populations, differentiated by behaviours and attitudes. Healthful adults, healthful young adults, healthful talkers and young athletes were classed as health-orientated clusters. Unhealthful adults, unhealthful young adults and worried older adults were described as unhealthy clusters. Unhealthful adults were unconcerned about their health and were unwilling to change. Accordingly, the authors suggested the need for a campaign which focused on changing perceived social norms and providing cues and incentives in the physical environment. Unhealthful young adults were unconcerned but ill-informed and they suggested the need for an awareness raising campaign. Finally, the worried older adult had high anxiety about their health but lacked the knowledge, self-efficacy and social support to change behaviours. For this group, initiatives that increased awareness, self-efficacy and social reinforcement in the community were likely to maximize the effect of any initiative.

Exchange theory states that products and services within the marketplace are bought and sold at acceptable costs and benefits for both buyer and seller. Although possibly the most controversial aspect of social marketing (see Buchanan et al. 1994), it suggests that if health promotion can demonstrate to the 'buyer' that the perceived benefits (improved health, social status, and so on) of an innovation outweigh its costs (deviation from social norms, financial, and so on) then it is more likely to be adopted. In this, the model appears to be an economic analogue of the health belief and protection motivation theories. A consumer orientation refers to a population's involvement in all aspects of a health promotion initiative. This entails not only an assessment of a population's needs, which can include recipient variables such as issue involvement, self-efficacy and perceived norms, but monitoring recipients' responses to campaigns and adapting them accordingly.

The concern with the consumer naturally leads to a research strategy based on audience segmentation and formative research. Audience segmentation is a process through which heterogeneous populations are divided into smaller homogeneous groups. Typically, the dimensions used for segmentation have been demographic and behavioural. However, there has been an increasing recognition that recipient cognitions such as information avoidance and perceived risk are also important (see above; Slater and Flora 1991). Formative research covers a broad range of activities but has been operationalized as concept development, message development and message testing (Maibach 1993). Observation, focus groups, and in-depth interviewing are used to develop relevant message content. Finally, channel analysis compares the effectiveness of any particular media channel (television, radio, leaflets etc.) in accessing both the general population (its reach), and the specific population to whom the content is addressed (its specificity).

The result of such research is a marketing mix which establishes the appropriate product, price, place, promotion, positioning and politics. The product is the intervention, health behaviour or relevant psychological target construct. This needs to have an identifiable brand name or image. The price refers to any cost, be it monetary, psychological or social, involved with the adoption or use of the product. At the individual level, successful interventions are likely to be those that reduce costs by suggesting small steps in behaviour change and increase rewards by offering immediate benefits. At the environmental level, easy access and reduced monetary costs can also help to market new behaviours. These commercial constructs clearly reflect the theories of social learning, the health belief model and protection motivation theory.

The place is the distribution point for, or availability of, the product, the most important factor being ease of access. This may be influenced by the chosen channel of media communication, such as leaflets or videos or the positioning of a television campaign. It may involve environmental manipulations, such as healthy eating policies or increasing the availability of low or non-alcoholic drinks. Promotion involves informing or persuading people of the utility of the product. Attention here is given particularly to the source and content of any message.

Positioning refers to the niche target group for the product, including demographics, behaviour of cognitions. In the past the tendency has been to concentrate on demographics, but Winett (1995) argues that psychological theories such as stages of change theory (Prochaska and DiClemente 1984) could be used to inform positioning. Finally, politics refers to the economic and social environment in which the product is sold. This recognizes that the economic, political, social and physical environment exert an influence on the individual, and that health promotion initiatives may be ineffective if attempts at facilitating behavioural change are not viewed within this context.

Understanding social processes in communities

Results obtained from persuasion studies in the laboratory have informed the design of campaigns in the community. However, evaluations of these campaigns have rarely compared the relative effectiveness of differing media content. Instead, they have typically focused on attitudinal and behavioural change within the target population consequent to media campaigns employing a number of differing media channels. Such an approach makes it difficult to disentangle the elements that make up a successful health promotion initiative in the community. However, understanding communication within communities may help us to understand the processes involved in responses to campaigns.

Television has been the prime channel of communication in general population approaches, and has been consistently shown to reinforce existing behaviour, raise awareness and set agendas, but have little or no effect on behaviour (Liebert and Schwertzenberg 1977; Lau *et al.* 1980; Wallack 1980). This failure to facilitate behavioural change has been found for behaviours as diverse as alcohol misuse (Blane and Hewitt 1977), seat-belt use (Robertson 1976), smoking (O'Keefe 1971; Flay 1987) and drink-driving (Cameron 1978). Accordingly, while television and other mass media may impact on a large audience, they have low specificity and low influence (Chaffe and Mutz 1988). Although specificity can be increased by proper placement, it has been argued that television campaigns are only likely to succeed if they achieve monopolization, channelling and supplementation (Lazarfield and Merton 1972).

Monopolization requires audiences to receive a single point of view and no counter-argument, such as advertising that stresses the attractiveness of high fat foods. Although attempts can be made to reduce counter-messages by restricting advertising of unhealthy products and reducing portrayals of unhealthy behaviours in the media, monopolization is an unrealistic goal. Channelling refers to attempts to manipulate existing cognitions rather than creating new ones, for example by providing relevant information to those already wishing to quit smoking. Finally, supplementation refers to the provision of complementary activity to support messages, for example by providing advice lines, smoking cessation groups, developing appropriate environmental policies, and so on.

An important determinant of the success of any media campaign is its dissemination through the population as a result of interpersonal communication (Rogers 1983). Smokers, for example, who discussed a campaign were more likely to succeed in cessation attempts (Puska *et al.* 1985; Jason *et al.* 1987). However, it is unclear whether discussion was a result of the campaign or as a consequence of the pre-existing salience of the issue to the individual. While such communication may occur naturally, it may also be manipulated by health promotion programmes. In North Karelia, doctors identified as opinion leaders were asked to promote appropriate behavioural change. In the Stanford project (see Chapter 7, pages 120–2), a number of people found to be within the ninetieth percentile of risk for CHD were identified, received counselling in behaviour change techniques, and were then asked to promote such changes among friends and colleagues. Each person reported discussing health-related issues with, on average, six other people. Discussion can also increase agenda setting among key gate-keepers of the media and policy.

Interpersonal networks have also been utilized by health promoters and school educators. Parcel *et al.* (1989), for example, described how diffusion strategies were used to influence the adoption of the Minnesota Smoking

Prevention Programme, an innovative peer-led approach to smoking prevention, within schools. Three aspects of diffusion theory were used. First, the benefits and ease of use of the package were emphasized through the use of a video demonstrating its effect in the classroom and pupils' positive reaction to the programme. Second, teachers considered to be opinion leaders were invited to a workshop on the programme and asked to disseminate the video to their colleagues. Finally, a newsletter advocating the benefits of the programme was mailed to all the workshop attenders and their colleagues in an attempt to use the local informational networks. Macdonald (1992) provided a similar description of the diffusion of the *Working with Groups* packages designed for health promotion specialists in the early 1980s. The package was designed to be easily used and understood and workshops were run for early adopters. Regional coordinators were recruited to disseminate the package and instruct other trainers; they also acted as an effective informational social network. Diffusion followed the classic S-shaped curve. By 1986 all regions in the UK had been exposed to the package and over 700 people had participated in training workshops before going on, in turn, to run their own workshops.

Summary and conclusions

Research conducted on attitude change in the laboratory, although subject to validity problems, has highlighted the importance of understanding the interaction of source, content and receiver variables in responses to media messages. Results have provided a frequently contradictory and often confusing picture. However, models such as the elaboration likelihood model have provided some explanation of possible psychological processes. Their utility for health promotion may be to focus media campaigns away from mass to more targeted approaches, and to increase research examining how messages are received and integrated into existing cognitions. Outside the laboratory the majority of research has failed to adequately explain why campaigns succeed or not. There is, therefore, a need to understand how media messages are disseminated and interpreted through existing social systems. Both social marketing and diffusion theory, although open to criticism, may provide a framework to examine these processes.

Suggested reading

Lau, R., Kane, R., Berry, S., Ware, J. and Roy, D. (1980) Channeling health: a review of the evaluation of televised health campaigns. *Health Education Quarterly*, 7: 56–87.

O'Keefe, D. (1990) *Persuasion: Theory and Research*. Newbury Park, CA: Sage.

Wallack, L. (1981) Mass media campaigns: the odds against finding behavior change. *Health Education Quarterly*, 1: 209–60.

Population based interventions

Health promotion initiatives targeted at large populations probably form the most cost-effective approach to health promotion. In previous chapters, we have reviewed how psychological theory may inform interventions at a number of levels. Social cognition theories, such as the theory of planned behaviour (Ajzen 1985) and social learning (Bandura 1977) provide general theories of behavioural decision-making. Others, such as the health belief model (Becker 1974) and protection motivation theory (Maddux and Rogers 1983) provide more health or threat-specific explanatory models. Diffusion theory (Rogers 1983) informs our understanding of how individuals within society react to and disseminate health messages. None of the theories alone provides a full understanding of the processes underlying the uptake and maintenance of new health behaviours. Together, however, they suggest key variables and processes that may interact to predict behaviour and which can provide the bases to any health promotion initiative targeted at behavioural change.

When discussing these theories we have done so either in the context of a purely theoretical review or studies where they have been tested in the field, usually under tightly controlled conditions where the impact of specific experimental manipulations can be measured. In this chapter we extend this discussion by examining how social cognition models have informed the design and implementation of some of the most elaborate health promotion initiatives so far conducted, focusing on large-scale health promotion initiatives in the workplace and wider community. Of importance is that the initiatives suggested by the theories, when used imaginatively, incorporate interventions targeted both at the individual and the wider environment.

Worksite health promotion

In the United States, improving the health of the workforce has implications not only for the well-being of employees, but has resulted in less sick leave, accidents at work, and employer health insurance costs (Pelletier 1993). These have proven powerful incentives to large scale employers, and many now conduct health promotion programmes to actively promote the health of their workers. These may involve environmental measures such as providing 'no smoking' areas or healthy diet options. More active programmes have involved health screening programmes and incentive schemes to foster change.

There are a number of advantages and disadvantages associated with the use of the worksite for health promotion initiatives. From the employees' perspective, they are convenient and relatively cheap. In addition, they provide the opportunity for social support and the opportunity to participate with friends and co-workers. These strengths may also be disadvantages; the timing of meetings may interfere with other valued activities and individuals may not wish to disclose some behaviours in front of their peers. If not handled appropriately, such programmes may also lead workers to feel coerced by management to participate. Individually targeted programmes may also foster resentment in those who do not receive them. For employers, potential benefits include better employee morale and public relations (Everly and Feldman 1985; Cataldo and Coates 1986) as well as reduced health care costs, particularly in the USA (e.g. Harvey *et al.* 1993), and reduced absenteeism (Bertera 1990). In contrast, as many programmes focus on individuals rather than organizational structures, there is a danger of victim blaming and developing ineffective programmes.

From a theoretical perspective, the worksite offers an excellent opportunity to maximize behavioural change through long-term individual programmes, and the potential for environmental policies and manipulations to foster and maintain such change. However not all programmes have utilized the full potential of the worksite. A number of worksites have provided health screening clinics similar to those conducted in primary care settings, with no provision for follow-up or support through other environmental changes. These gain no advantage over similar interventions conducted in other settings. Rose *et al.* (1980), for example, reported five-year smoking cessation rates of 7 per cent in a group of workers who received a follow-up of four consultations by company physicians following screening. Among those who only participated in the screening process, there was no reduction in smoking level. More success was reported by Shipley *et al.* (1988). Their findings indicated two-year cessation rates of 23 per cent among those who received screening plus counselling and 17 per cent of those who received screening alone as part of the Johnson & Johnson 'Live for Life' programme. Both cessation rates are high, and those of the screening-only group are significantly higher than those typically found following screening only. However, even in this context, the extended programme proved more effective than screening alone.

Not only is screening less effective than more complex or supportive interventions, it also attracts fewer participants. Erfurt *et al.* (1990), for example, compared the uptake for three programmes conducted at separate worksites offering screening alone, in combination with health education classes, and a 'high intensity programme'. This involved screening and health education classes in addition to environmental changes including establishing buddy systems, competitions, and increased exercise facilities at the plant. About half those eligible participated in the two major programmes of weight loss and smoking cessation offered by the high intensity programme. This compares with participation rates of less than 10 per cent in the site offering only health education classes and less than 1 per cent in the screening-only site. Accordingly, while the worksite provides an excellent setting for health promotion, its benefits can only be maximized through programmes which utilize its environmental and social resources to the full. The next section of the chapter examines the impact of programmes which have adopted such policies.

Reducing risk for CHD

Incentive-based approaches

The worksite provides an opportunity to manipulate the gains associated with behavioural change (Bandura 1977). Some programmes, such as Employee Assistance Programmes (Cyster and McEwan 1988) work on a process of negative reinforcement. Typically targeted at those whose behaviour is adversely affecting their job performance, changes in behaviour are rewarded by not losing one's job. Fortunately, initiatives targeted at the wider workforce have been more positively oriented and have provided incentives as a reward for positive behavioural change.

An example of such an initiative is provided by Klesges et al. (1986). They reported the outcome of a quit-smoking competition conducted in five workplaces. All sites received a six-week cognitive behavioural programme focusing on cessation skills. In addition, enrolees in four of the five sites participated in competing teams; participants at the fifth site acted as a control condition. By the end of the programme, 31 per cent of participants in the control site and 22 per cent of those in the competing sites had stopped smoking. At the six-month follow-up, the cessation rates were 18 and 14 per cent respectively – a modest advantage favouring the control group. However, 88 per cent of smoking employees at the competition sites joined the programme in comparison to 54 per cent of smokers at the control site. The differential recruitment rate resulted in a 16 per cent reduction in the number of smokers at the competition sites, in contrast to a 7 per cent reduction in the group-only sites.

Another large-scale incentive-based programme of a very different nature was reported by Jeffery et al. (1993). They randomly allocated 32 worksites to receive either a two-year-long extended health education programme or to act as a control. The programme comprised bi-annual health education courses, each lasting 22 weeks. Classes provided training in cognitive-behavioural strategies for smoking and weight loss. In addition, participants selected an amount of money to be deducted from their pay, with refunds for weight loss and smoking cessation. Recruitment was through direct invitation and advertising through the worksite. Weight losses in the intervention sites averaged 4.8 lbs, and 43 per cent of smoking participants quit. However, as only 12 per cent of eligible smokers participated in the programme, the net gain within the workplace for smoking cessation was about 3 per cent. No between-site differences were found for weight loss. Comparison of these results with those of Klesges and colleagues (1986) described above suggests that employees prefer schemes that reward success, not punish failure.

A lower cost intervention was reported by Glasgow et al. (1993), in which an incentive scheme for smoking cessation was combined with individual monthly meetings with research staff who monitored breath carbon monoxide levels and encouraged change, but did not provide 'expert' advice. Abstinent smokers were eligible for monthly lottery prizes. Nineteen per cent of workers who smoked participated in the study. At the time of the final lottery draw, one year into the programme, 20 per cent of this group were no longer smoking. These results compare well with those of screening programmes and self-help interventions and suggest that relatively simple incentive-based initiatives may facilitate smoking cessation. However, the reliability of these results is compromised by the lack of a control group.

Phased interventions

An interesting project was reported by Thompson et al. (1995) in which they targeted smokers, identified through a health survey, with a 'stepped model of care' lasting for up to one and a half years. Telephone contacts every three months provided motivational messages tailored to the individual's stage of cessation, and guidance on how best to quit should they choose to. Subsequent, more intensive interventions, included the provision of self-help manuals and referrals to formal quit programmes. Participants could withdraw from the scheme should they choose at any time during the course of the study. Not surprisingly, perhaps, participation rates fell during the course of the study, although at worst 60 per cent of those still smoking agreed to continue in the programme. Self-report data suggested that 18 per cent of all the smokers identified quit smoking, while 16 per cent abstained for a period of six months or more. However, given the somewhat coercive nature of the programme, in the absence of corroborative evidence these data should perhaps be considered with some caution.

Facilitating social support

Social support can be a powerful facilitator of behavioural change. It reflects social norms which support change and provides the opportunity for mutual help in achieving desired goals. In a naturalistic study of the relationship between social support, levels of engagement in health-enhancing behaviours, and attempts at behavioural change, Terborg *et al.* (1995) measured individual's perceptions of the social support available from management and colleagues for their not smoking or having a low cholesterol diet. Their results indicated a modest but significant association between perceived support and healthy behaviour at baseline. However, this measure did not predict future cessation attempts or changes in cholesterol levels during the subsequent intervention phase of the Take Heart project (see below).

However, where social support has been actively manipulated some gains have been reported. The incentive approach of Klesges *et al.* (1986) provides one successful example of this approach. Similarly, Brownell and Felix (1987) manipulated social support through the development of teams in an attempt to increase participation and adherence to a weight reduction programme. Participants were organized into competitive teams, given relevant self-help manuals and a baseline weight assessment conducted. Throughout the programme, the results from weekly weigh-ins were displayed in a prominent position at each worksite. After approximately 15 weeks, attrition was less than 1 per cent and average weight loss was 5.5 kg – a substantial success for a weight loss programme. In the context of smoking cessation, Jason *et al.* 1987 assigned 425 workers in 43 worksites to a media presentation alone or in combination with the provision of six 45-minute support group meetings. These were not intended as a means of providing 'expert' help or advice. Rather, they provided a forum for those on the programme to gain mutual support from their fellow sufferers. Results indicated that the combined condition yielded superior self-report cessation rates both immediately post-intervention (41 versus 21 per cent) and at the three-month follow-up (22 versus 12 per cent).

Lifestyle interventions

One of the most substantial and careful worksite health promotion initiatives so far conducted was reported by Glasgow *et al.* (1995). In the Take Heart programme, conducted in 26 worksites in Oregon, all members of the workforce were invited to attend health screening, including biochemical and behavioural measures. An average of 48 per cent of the workforce took part in the survey. Half the worksites then engaged in an 18-month intervention, involving a variety of environmental, educational, and skills-based interventions in an attempt to modify workers' dietary and smoking habits. Half acted as control sites. Interventions were selected to maximize effects in employees at each stage of the process of change. Smoking interventions included the provision of self-help kits and group support meetings. Dietary interventions included written materials, presentations with food samples, and cooking demonstrations. Policy issues included the provision of 'no smoking' areas, increasing healthy food options in the cafeterias and vending machines, and stopping the sale of tobacco on-site. Their results were disappointing. After one and a half years of this programme, no between-site differences were found on measures of smoking prevalence, dietary fat intake and serum cholesterol. The authors' 'inescapable' conclusion was that the Take Heart project did not improve employee health behaviours related to nutrition and tobacco use more than did repeated measures alone.

This somewhat disappointing result is not unique. Other large-scale projects (Jacobs et al. 1986; COMMIT Research Group 1995) have apparently failed to facilitate more behavioural change than that in comparison areas. In a somewhat obtuse manner, this may actually reflect the success of health promotion. In each case, the data do not suggest that health promotion initiatives did not facilitate behavioural change; rather, these changes were no greater than those which occurred in the wider population. We therefore have to consider why these wider population changes are occurring. One hypothesis, to which we return below, is that they too are occurring as a response to changing population norms and diffused health education messages, such as those we increasingly encounter in magazines, foodstores, and a variety of other settings. These may not form part of any formal health promotion programme. However, they do reflect the increasing interest in health and health maintenance engendered by more formal health-promotion programmes, and form a backdrop against which any formal programme will necessarily be compared.

Reducing risk for cancer

Combining education and cues to healthy behaviour

While weight loss programmes may involve reduced fat consumption, few studies have examined the effect of programmes targeted at facilitating dietary change in fat and other nutrients to reduce the risk of cancer. The Treatwell Program (Sorensen et al. 1992; Hebert et al. 1993) was one of those infrequent initiatives. This established a programme providing classes and food demonstrations for the workforce. These were augmented by food labelling in worksite cafeterias. The goal of the programme was to reduce dietary fat to 30 per cent of total calories and to increase dietary fibre to between 20 and 30 grams per day. The intervention lasted a period of 15 months, and changes in diet following the programme were compared with those of a control worksite which did not receive it. By this time, modest but clinically insignificant reductions in fat consumption were found among participants in the active condition. There was no evidence of changes in consumption of dietary fibre. However, reductions in consumption of carotene, thought to be involved in epithelial cancer, favouring the intervention group were found. The authors suggest that some of their negative findings may stem from relatively insensitive methods of measuring intake. Nevertheless, the overall impact of the intervention on risk for cancer was negligible (Hebert *et al.* 1993).

A European approach

Changing the work environment

The vast majority of worksite interventions in the USA have involved attempts to modify lifestyle factors, primarily through the provision of screening services and less frequently through more extended initiatives. While clearly of benefit, this approach implicitly places the responsibility for workers' health on the individual. Worksite health promotion is much less established in Europe and other areas than in the USA. However, this lack of a strong history may permit differing, and perhaps more innovative, types of intervention. One such was reported by Maes *et al.* (in submission). Their intervention, conducted at a Dutch worksite focused both on lifestyle change, and also modifying key aspects of the working environment in order to foster mental and physical well-being throughout the workforce – a sharp contrast to the American model of disease prevention.

The first year of the programme focused on behavioural change, by establishing lunchtime health education classes and exercise programmes. In the second and third years, the programme became more innovative. Maes's team drew upon a substantial literature which has identified the optimal working conditions within the workplace, including individuals working within their capabilities, avoiding short and repetitive performance tasks, having some control over the organization of their own work, sufficient social contact, and feeling involved in the company. Over the course of this second phase they attempted, within the constraints of production, to permit each individual to work in conditions as close to these ideals as possible. In addition, they provided training in communication and leadership skills for managers and identified methods through which they could recognize, prevent and reduce stress within the workforce.

Four groups of workers were followed for the duration of the programme: those working in the intervention worksite, those in the control sites, and participants and non-participants in the individual lifestyle-change programme. The programme effects seem specific to the interventions conducted. By the end of the individual intervention phase, participants in the lifestyle programme evidenced greater reductions in risk for CHD than those of the control group, as well as lower levels of depression and hostility. By the end of the third year of the project, these gains were no longer evident. However, the wider intervention was associated with increased quality of work and lower absenteeism rates in comparison to the control sites over the duration of the intervention.

Community-based programmes

Reducing risk for CHD

Coronary heart disease (CHD) remains the leading cause of premature morbidity in western countries; risk is also primarily mediated by modifiable, behavioural, factors. Accordingly, much of the effort invested in disease prevention has focused on CHD, through a series of large scale evaluated interventions in the USA and Europe (see Smith *et al.* 1994). These have attempted to determine what our best technology of change can achieve, and relied on expert staff and large budgets. More recently cheaper, simpler, and perhaps more cost-effective, interventions have been conducted and evaluated (e.g. Fries *et al.* 1992; Goodman *et al.* 1995). Rather than review all these projects, space limitations dictate that we examine the effectiveness of a representative sample. This means, necessarily, that some important programmes (e.g. the Pawtucket Heart Health Program; Carleton *et al.* 1995) are not described here. However, the findings we report are typical.

The Stanford Projects

The Stanford Three Towns Project (Farquhar *et al.* 1977) was one of the first substantial community heart disease prevention projects. Explicitly based on social learning theory principles, it explored the impact of media-based and individual programmes on risk for CHD in both the general population and those at high risk for disease. It involved three communities: Tracey, Gilroy and Watsonville. Tracey acted as a control area and received no intervention. Gilroy and Watsonville received an intensive year-long media-based intervention followed by a repeated, less intensive, intervention. In addition, a sample of Watsonville residents at high risk for CHD participated with their partners in a programme of 10 home and group counselling sessions. These individuals were asked to disseminate the knowledge they had gained at these sessions to friends and acquaintances. Accordingly, a hierarchy of expected change in levels of risk for CHD was expected: Tracey, Gilroy, and Watsonville.

   The media programme involved a series of stages: agenda setting, the provision of information, modelling change and skills for change, and finally 'cues to action'. In the case of smoking, for example, the media first provided information on the risks of smoking and the benefits of cessation. This was followed by information on how to quit. Televised smoking cessation groups provided models of behavioural change, intended to provide skills and increase self-efficacy judgements in smokers. To promote dietary change, the same sequence was followed: information on the benefits of dietary change, demonstration of different cooking techniques and distribution of recipe leaflets to all households, followed by prompts to maintain change through modelling enjoying healthy eating. The counselling programme involved a similar, skills-based, programme of change.

Risk for CHD was measured in samples representative of the general population and those at high risk for CHD. In the former, one-year follow-up measures revealed a reduction in risk relative to Tracey of 12 per cent in Gilroy and 21 per cent in Watsonville. These gains were maintained up to the final assessment two years later. In the high-risk samples, those who entered the individual intervention programme in Watsonville evidenced a 33 per cent reduction in risk relative to the equivalent Tracey group at one year, reducing to a 21 per cent reduction two years later. The gains in Gilroy were less spectacular but still significant, with reductions relative to Tracey of 15 per cent at year one, and 8 per cent at the three-year follow-up (Maccoby 1988). The methodology used to analyse the impact of the programme was subject to some criticism (see Kasl 1980; Leventhal et al. 1980; Meyer et al. 1980). Changes in risk for CHD, for example, were assessed by measuring changes in a cohort of individuals, selected at the outset of the project and subjected to repeat measures at each assessment time. This may have resulted in some reactive effects. There was some evidence, for example, that a small percentage of those in the intervention cohort modified their behaviour for a short period prior to assessment, a process which may have disproportionately increased the apparent effect of the intervention. Differential drop-out from this cohort in intervention and control areas may also have distorted their results. Nevertheless, these were generally viewed as indicative of the potentially powerful impact of community interventions.

The Stanford Five-City Project (Farquhar et al. 1990) began in 1978 and attempted to combine the previous methods of intervention with a higher level of community focus and to address larger population centres. Community-initiated collaborative teaching programmes, in particular, formed an important arm of the programme, and by its fifth year 27 per cent of those people who knew of the programme had been involved in these programmes. The intervention also attempted to modify environmental factors by, for example, encouraging shops and restaurants to provide healthy foodstuffs. The impact of the intervention in two cities was compared with changes in three control areas not receiving the intervention.

The outcome of the intervention was measured in two ways. First, by measuring changes in a cohort of individuals, selected at the outset of the project and subjected to repeat measures at each assessment time. Second, through the use of separate samples selected from the populations of each city at the time of assessment. Both were representative of the wider populations in the intervention and control communities. The use of separate samples reduced the risk of reactive effects as may have occurred in the Three Communities Study. However, it may provide a more conservative estimate of change, and be affected by other biases. For example, as the samples are representative of the population at the time the measures are taken, changing population demographics may change the prevalence of risk factors measured over time, regardless of any behavioural changes engaged in by the community. Accordingly, both types of assessment have problems of interpretation. However, as both methods are subject to different biases, consistent findings from both methods may provide evidence of considerable strength. There is also the potential that two sets of outcome measures may give conflicting results, as indeed they did for the Stanford Study.

In a cohort followed for the duration of the study, knowledge of CHD risk factors rose in all samples but more in the intervention areas. Measures of some risk factors, notably total cholesterol, resting pulse and body-mass index, fell more in the intervention areas at the beginning of the project, but by the end did not differ significantly from the control area (e.g. Fortmann *et al.* 1993). Only blood pressure and smoking rates differed at the end of the intervention. Nevertheless, risk for CHD was lowered by 16 per cent in the intervention population cohort in contrast to 3 per cent in those of the control cities. In a series of cross-sectional surveys conducted over the period of the project, smoking rates did not differ between the intervention and control cities at any time. This was reflected in CHD risk scores, which fell in the intervention area by 16 per cent and in the control area by 14 per cent, a non-significant difference. More positively, those who were at high risk for CHD evidenced the greatest behavioural change – sufficient to result in significant reductions in mortality (Farquhar *et al.* 1990).

The North Karelia Project

The North Karelia Project coincided with the Stanford Projects, and involved some of the team from Stanford. Not surprisingly, the interventions have a common theoretical basis, with the contribution of social learning theory, the theory of reasoned action, and McGuire's model of persuasive communication specifically cited. Media interventions were staged as in Stanford, and involved models of change. However, more attention was given to changing social norms, which previously had supported a high cholesterol diet. Classes were made available locally to teach, for example, new cooking methods and to help people quit smoking.

The North Karelia Project differed significantly from its American counterpart in its emphasis on environmental manipulations. It worked with local food manufacturers and distributors to produce and promote low fat meat and dairy products. Environmental contingencies were also established to promote behavioural change, through the development of healthy restaurants and 'no smoking' areas. Using the principles of diffusion, the project utilized volunteer lay leaders, identified through informal interviews with local people who were trained to act as models and educators. This simple process has many advantages. Lay leaders provide information and skills from a respected source, model appropriate behaviour change, and serve to modify perceived behavioural norms. In addition to attempts at facilitating individual behavioural change, screening services were established to identify and treat hypertension. Over the first five years of the project 14,000 blood pressures were recorded in screening clinics.

Evaluation of the project involved comparisons with an adjacent county on measures of coronary risk at five and 10 years into the project. Evidence of significant reductions in most risk factors for coronary heart disease within North Karelia was found at each assessment. However, these were generally matched by gains in the comparison area. In addition, smoking levels among women actually rose in the project area during the life of the project. These, and some other issues led one of the principal investigators (Salonen 1987) to suggest that while the Karelia Project had demonstrated the logistical possibility of running such a project, the case for the effect-iveness of such projects in changing behaviour and coronary risk remained unproven.

The Minnesota Heart Health Program

The Minnesota Heart Health Program (MHHP; Jacobs *et al.* 1986) provides a further example of an intervention focusing on both community and professional involvement. This comprised a five-year intervention based on social learning theory, persuasive-communications theory, and involve-ment of community leaders and institutions. In the community, activities were guided by a community advisory board made up of influential political, business, health and other community leaders. This choice of authority figures is interesting, as they involved people who could direct policy, for example in the workplace, rather than act as individual role models as in the North Karelia Project. The mass media was used to promote awareness of the programme and to reinforce other educational components. However, less emphasis appears to have been placed on using it as a means of education through modelling change than the Stanford Projects. In contrast, the MHHP focused on individual screening in primary care and direct contact with indi-viduals through competitions, telephone support, classes in the community and worksite, self-help materials, and home correspondence programmes. In addition, the programme manipulated the environment to facilitate and maintain change, for example, through food labelling, healthy menus in restaurants, and increasing opportunities for physical recreation.

The programme targeted change on key CHD risk factors including smok-ing, low levels of exercise, and raised blood pressure and serum cholesterol levels. Interventions targeted at smoking included supportive telephone calls, worksite quit classes, home correspondence courses, and worksite manipula-tions including increased smoke-free areas. Additional community-based programmes involved quit and win competitions, in which smokers entered their name into a series of prize draws in which they could win prizes if their name was drawn and they were not smoking at the time. The effect of these interventions is reported by Lando *et al.* (1995). Quit and win contests achieved an approximate 5 per cent take-up, with quit rates in the early competitions approximating 20 per cent; the impact was less in later competitions. Classes achieved a quit rate of about 13 per cent, with slightly lower success rates for correspondence courses. Worksite intervention led to increased adoption of restrictive policies throughout Minnesota, although only 9 per cent of worksites participated in the project.

Despite these findings, there was little evidence to suggest any substantial differences in levels of smoking cessation between intervention and control areas, and the researchers admitted that the impact of the programme was only marginal at best. They suggested that this relative lack of impact, in comparison with the early Stanford Project, reflected an acceleration in secular changes in smoking level over the period of time between the two projects. The MHHP is not alone in these findings. Two major trials in the USA (COMMIT Research Group 1995) and The Netherlands (Mudde *et al.* 1995) reported no greater changes than secular trends in their intervention areas following sophisticated smoking cessation interventions, even when those in the intervention groups were given a choice of interventions in which they could participate (Mudde *et al.* 1995).

Initiatives targeted at reducing obesity included adult education classes for weight control, exercise, and cholesterol, a worksite weight control programme, and a home correspondence course for weight loss and a weight gain prevention programme. The latter involved a year-long programme consisting of three components: a regular newsletter, weight control classes, and a financial incentive for weight control. Unfortunately for the programme, the most dramatic finding was one of increasing weight over time. Between the beginning of the trial and its end, the average weight of an adult in the communities increased by nearly 7 lb – a finding mirrored in a cohort who were known to have taken part in the activities of the MHHP. The author of the report (Jeffery 1995: 286) concluded that 'the MHHP had little or no effect on levels of obesity'.

More specific community interventions

Reducing risk for cancer

Population level interventions targeted specifically at the reduction of risk for cancer are much less common than those targeted at CHD. One such, was the 'five a day – for better health' programme of California (Foerster *et al.* 1995). This 18-month-long intervention utilized the strategies considered successful in the CHD programmes: mass media, health education and community organization. The goal was to encourage people to eat five servings of fruit and vegetables each day, and to educate the population about the link between a poor diet and cancer. Over the period of the programme there was a significant rise in levels of knowledge concerning the diet–cancer link. Those who identified a low fruit and vegetable diet being linked to cancer increased from 24 to 32 per cent. The percentage of adults who said they should eat more fruit and vegetables rose from 52 to 60. However, fruit and vegetable consumption rose by only 1.3 per cent – a figure no different to long term trends in the wider population.

Reducing risk for HIV transmission

Reducing risk for HIV transmission presents a number of challenges for health promotion. Public sensibilities may prevent explicitly sexual material being broadcast on the media. Embarrassment and fear of stigmatization may inhibit attendance at open education meetings or counselling sessions (Smith 1987). Conversely, some gay men's fear of prejudice when being counselled in medical settings may interfere with the counselling process (Ostrow 1984). As a consequence, interventions to reduce the spread of HIV have perhaps been some of the most innovative yet used by health promoters. Interventions have been conducted in individuals' homes, in home parties and in gay bars and bathhouses (Mantell *et al*. 1987). They have involved outreach workers working with prostitutes (Blakey and Frankland 1995) in the context of sexually transmitted disease (Kolata 1987) and in drug users' clinics (Malow *et al*. 1994). They have involved individual or group work utilizing workshop methods and erotic material (Robert and Rosser 1990: Tudiver *et al*. 1992).

Unfortunately, from a research perspective, ethical considerations often prevent comparisons of the effectiveness of any intervention against a no treatment group (to withhold a potentially effective intervention from a group at significant risk of disease is ethically questionable). In addition, many of these interventions are funded by local health and social services, for whom research is not a priority. As a consequence, many of these interventions have not been formally assessed (e.g. Mantell *et al*. 1987). Nevertheless, perhaps reflecting the health imperatives associated with HIV infection, these interventions have reached a wider range of racial, economic, and educational backgrounds than many other approaches (Mantell *et al*. 1987).

Perhaps the most effective series of interventions were those conducted in the epicentre of the epidemic: San Francisco. Between 1985 and 1988 the number of individuals engaging in unprotected anal intercourse among the gay population fell from 36 to 3 per cent (Coates 1990). The reasons for these behavioural changes are multiple and it has proven impossible to determine all the influences on behaviour. Seroprevalence levels of 50 per cent, the associated high risk of infection, and the high probability of individuals knowing someone with AIDS must clearly have affected behaviour.

Some behavioural change may also be attributable to health promotion initiatives running throughout this period (McKusick *et al*. 1985). The San Francisco programme was based on the three principles: increasing individuals' personal threat of HIV infection, reducing the barriers to safe sex through messages of how it may be enjoyed and skills training, and modification of peer norms. Media campaigns, targeted at specific and general populations, gave information on the health risks associated with certain behaviours. They were also used to teach safer sex and negotiation skills, and to provide information about prevailing and desired community norms. Information provision and skills training also occurred through a variety of existing systems including schools, workplaces, health care systems, churches, clubs, and so on. This was combined with individual programmes with drug users, strengthening sexually transmitted disease programmes, and aggressive use of outreach to provide contraception to high-risk women. In addition, testing for HIV antibodies was made easily available, as were condoms, which were available in a variety of settings, including schools, pharmacies, hotels, and toilets. The media were used to make people aware of the availability of condoms and to demonstrate their use.

A cohort of gay and bisexual men was followed over the first year of the project to assess its impact on behaviour and attitudes. At baseline, 60 per cent reported engaging in high-risk sexual behaviour; 50 per cent of this group reported engaging in unprotected anal intercourse. One year later, 30 per cent reported engaging in high-risk behaviour, of whom 12 per cent reported incidents of unprotected anal intercourse. Predictors of change included knowledge of personal HIV status, self-efficacy judgements concerning safe sex, and the perception of peer norms as supportive of safer sex practices.

Summary and conclusions

At first glance, the effectiveness of population interventions in reducing the incidence of disease appears disappointing. Early CHD prevention projects, whether at the worksite or in the wider community, evidenced significant reductions in the prevalence of risk factors in comparison to control areas. Later projects have appeared less successful. Against this background, some commentators (e.g. Pelletier 1993) remain strong advocates of the effectiveness of population approaches to health promotion; others (e.g. Smith et al. 1994) are more cautious in their claims.

Given the theoretical and practical complexity, not to mention cost, of these programmes these results may be considered disappointing. However, as we noted before they may actually represent a success story. At worst, health promotion activities have not failed to facilitate behavioural change; rather, these changes were no greater than those which occurred in the wider population. We therefore have to consider why these wider population changes are occurring. One strong hypothesis is that they too are occurring as a response to diffused health education messages, and changing secular norms. These may occur in response to any formal health promotion programme. However, they do reflect the increasing interest in health and healthy lifestyles engendered by more formal health promotion programmes, and form a backdrop against which any formal programme will necessarily be compared.

In addition, comparison areas may themselves be engaged in health promotion activities. Heartbeat Wales affords an example of how these processes may reduce the apparent impact of a large-scale health promotion intervention. Between 1985 and 1990, Heartbeat Wales formed a community heart disease prevention programme targeted at the adult population of Wales. Its evaluation strategy involved comparisons with a reference sample drawn from a matched region in England (Nutbeam *et al.* 1993). Over the course of its five-year intervention phase, although the Welsh samples evidenced significant behavioural changes these did not differ from those reported by the comparison group. A retrospective analysis of health promotion activity in the control area provided some clues as to why this was the case. Essentially, the level of health promotion activity in the area had matched that occurring in Wales. Some innovations piloted in Wales (food labelling and the Heartbeat Awards for caterers) had been adopted as part of the local health promotion strategy. In addition, a nationally funded programme (Look After Your Heart) mirrored many of the strategies of the Welsh programme in England.

The pervasive nature of health promotion, be it of a formal or informal nature, and the reducing prevalence of risk factors for many behaviourally mediated diseases, and disease rates themselves, is not coincidental. Community interventions have worked, albeit through wider channels than first envisaged. With this success in mind, we would argue that psychological theory has proved of value in the development of successful attempts at motivating and maintaining behavioural change within the wider community. However, the plateau that this form of intervention has reached suggests that future health promotion initiatives may usefully change in focus: either in terms of their target behaviours, or by moving from population programmes which still predominantly entail individual behavioural change to those involving more structural changes.

Suggested reading

Pelletier, K.R. (1993) A review and analysis of the health and cost-effective outcome studies of comprehensive health promotion and disease prevention programs at the worksite: 1991–1993 update. *American Journal of Health Promotion*, 8: 50–62.

Smith, C., Moore, L. and Trickey, H. (1994) *Community-Based Cardiovascular Disease Prevention: A Review of the Effectiveness of Health Education and Health Promotion.* Utrecht: International Union for Health Promotion and Health Education.

Tonnes, K. and Tilford, S. (1994) *Health Education: Effectiveness, Efficiency and Equity.* (2nd edn) London: Chapman and Hall.

Winnett, R.A., King, A.C. and Altman, D.G. (1989) *Health Psychology and Public Health. An Integrative Approach.* New York: Pergamon.

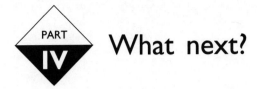

PART IV

What next?

Some final considerations

In earlier chapters we briefly considered how the social and environmental context in which we live impacts on health, and the corollary of this argument: that reducing population levels of ill-health requires both wide-ranging environmental change and individual behavioural change. In this chapter we examine these propositions further. In the first section, we return to examine the interrelationships between behavioural and structural models of health and health behaviour, focusing on issues of class and ethnicity. We then introduce a theory, known as symbolic interactionism (Mead 1934). This provides one understanding of the process of reciprocal influence between the individual and others in their social environment which can moderate the uptake and maintenance of health-related behaviours. In particular, we examine how these processes operate within the family system and the importance of examining such processes within health promotion research. The chapter then focuses on the need for health promotion to move from a model dominated by disease prevention, to one of facilitating positive health.

Social contexts, behaviour and health

The wider environment and health

Some of the most important documents relating to health in Britain in the 1990s were published under the rubric of *The Health of the Nation* (Department of Health 1992). These identified the health needs of the population and where resources should be invested to enable these to be met. They also established health or behaviourally defined targets (e.g. reduction of the prevalence of cigarette smoking to no more than 20 per cent of the adult population by the year 2000) to be achieved over identified time periods. The documents adopted a strong medical perspective, and were disappointing in their failure to address wider environmental variables as either causes of illness or determinants of health-related behaviours. Health behaviours were viewed as largely autonomous and randomly distributed within society. Such an approach is at odds with developments in public health and health promotion. Here, there is increasing acknowledgement that unhealthy behaviour is frequently maintained by cultural and social processes and that attempts to influence health behaviour which ignore such processes will be largely unsuccessful (Herzlich 1973; Caplan 1993).

Until now, our understandings of behavioural and cultural processes on health have been informed by separate and distinct theories and research approaches (Murphy and Bennett 1994). Behavioural explanations have focused on the individual; structuralist explanations on the social conditions in which they live. However, a number of commentators have suggested that behaviour can no longer be examined outside its social context (Blaxter 1983; Blane 1985) and that there is a clear need to develop a theory that links both types of explanation (Townsend and Davidson 1988; Whitehead 1988). The interaction between these variables is complex and some theories which have attempted to link them have been criticized as inadequate (Blaxter and Paterson 1982; Pill and Stott 1985). Nevertheless, we attempt to draw links between the two approaches, here examining psychological mechanisms which may mediate the relationship between social class, ethnicity, and health.

Initial explanations of the association between low socio-economic status (SES) and poor health focused on either behavioural or social explanations. Behavioural explanations suggested that differential rates of morbidity and mortality were consequent to those in the lower socio-economic groups engaging in more health-damaging behaviours (e.g. Bennett et al. 1991a). Structural explanations have focused, for example, on differential access to health care provision. Not only are the poor more likely to receive fewer and lower quality health services (Aday 1975; Brotherston 1976), they may be further disadvantaged in that access to health care represents one of the few health-protective resources they have (Williams 1990). Environmental models have focused on the higher levels of pollution, industrial toxins, and poorer quality housing etc. which may be experienced by those in the lower socio-economic groups (Watt and Ecob, 1992).

These models have been proposed as distinct and separate pathways through which poor health is mediated. There are clear links between them, however. People occupying lower socio-economic groups certainly do engage in more health-damaging behaviours than the economically more advantaged (Thomas et al. 1992), although this does not fully explain their high morbidity and mortality rates (Marmot et al. 1984). However, this association between a poor life situation and higher levels of health damaging behaviours may not be coincidental. To quote the response of one participant in a study in which we were involved (Bremble et al. 1991): 'a wish to sustain life has to be coupled with a will towards life. If you don't like what you've got you won't try to keep it very long.' Access to health care facilities may in part be a function of geographical proximity; it may also be a function of communication skills and perceptions of empowerment, which are differentially distributed through society. Finally, poor housing may not simply involve damp and dirt; increasingly, those living in poor housing are subject to a number of other environmental processes, including noise pollution, a significant psychological stressor.

Stress may prove one of the more important mediators between SES and health. It is unequally distributed through society, and those in socially disadvantaged groups report more stressors, including everyday hassles, than individuals in socially advantaged groups (Myers *et al.* 1974). In addition, the less well-off have less control over their environment and personal resources to mediate the impact of such stresses (Sleutjes 1990). Social support, an important moderator of the stress process, is also frequently less available to individuals in the lower socio-economic groups than those more economically advantaged (Werner and Smith 1982). These processes may combine to produce perceptions of powerlessness, lack of control (Mirowsky and Ross 1986) and lack of personal value, acceptance, and worthiness (Antonovsky 1987). Each has been implicated in the development of both mental and physical ill-health problems (see Carroll *et al.* 1993).

Disentangling the various genetic, social and psychological factors which may contribute to differences in morbidity and mortality between ethnic groups has proven difficult. The high incidence of mental illness among African-Caribbeans living in the UK, for example, has variously been explained by theories focusing on genetics, economic deprivation, discrimination and service provision problems (Littlewood and Lipsedge 1988). Here we focus on two processes through which these differences may be mediated: the influence of specific cultural norms which may counter health promotion messages targeted at the wider population, and socio-economic disadvantage.

Significant differences in social norms relevant to health behaviours can be found in different cultures. Gudykunst *et al.* (1987), for example, argued that as a result of their socialization, members of non-western cultures living in the west frequently consider health risks as a concern for other groups in society only, and not their own ethnic group. As a consequence they may be less likely to engage in health protective behaviours. Pittman *et al.* (1992) have argued that African-Americans' responses to AIDS have been influenced by differential identity development, gender role socialization, attitudes to contraception and homosexuality as well as differences in communication networks. However, in emphasizing cultural explanations over materialist explanations there is a danger of victim-blaming and stereotyping. Douglas (1995) illustrates this by reference to the Department of Health's rickets campaign conducted in the UK in the 1970s. Campaigns aimed at the white population identified the problem as one of poverty, and messages concentrated on including common foods containing vitamin D in one's diet. The campaign aimed at Asians identified the problem as one of cultural preferences and practices, and its advice focused on changing from traditional diets to British diets.

Socio-economic explanations of health inequalities focus on many of the issues already identified, including problems of access to health care, environmental stress, poor social support, and feelings of lack of control may each contribute to poor health status (Gottlieb and Green 1984). Ethnic minorities experience more problems in gaining access to health services such as cancer screening and antenatal care (Doyle 1991; Narang and Murphy 1994), and have lower survival rates following diagnosis of cancer or AIDS, than their white counterparts (Haan and Kaplan 1986; Primm 1987). They are also more likely to experience environmental stressors such as poverty, poor housing, unemployment and poor working conditions and to have less resources to respond to them (Brown 1984; Robinson 1984). Experiences of discrimination and racial harassment provide further environmental stress and reduce access to resources (Kessler and Neighbors 1986). In addition, as those occupying lower socio-economic groups have been found to have less future expectancy of life and to lack feelings of self-control, ethnicity may interact with low socio-economic status to produce double discrimination and powerlessness in blacks (Sleutjes 1990).

With the exception of specific targeted projects, large-scale health promotion campaigns have typically failed to address issues of ethnicity, gender or class (Flora and Thorensen 1988). Further, Douglas (1995: 75) states that 'it is significant to note that nowhere in the literature examining the WHO strategy (Health for All) is any reference made to black and minority ethnic communities and migrant communities in Europe'. This is a serious failing and represents an important area for future development.

Symbolic interactionism and the micro-environment

So far we have examined the impact of disadvantage on health. We have argued that the high prevalence of environmental and social stressors consequent to occupying low socio-economic groups and membership of many ethnic minorities may impact both directly and indirectly on health status. The social context in which we live, however, does more than moderate the levels of environmental stresses we encounter or provide us with more or less opportunities to engage in health-promoting behaviours. It also provides the sources of social influence on behaviour. Behavioural choices are frequently the consequence of negotiations with those around us, the nature of which change over the lifecourse. These may involve people with whom we are geographically close, including family, friends, co-workers and those involved in similar pastimes. They may involve members of similar cultural groups. Even more widely, they may involve consideration of behaviours and behavioural norms established by the media. Such processes have yet to be fully considered by psychological theory. As Winett (1995: 348) states, psychologists have traditionally focused on cognition and behaviour as the figure, with environment often the distant amorphous ground (or context). A reversal of figure and ground is not suggested; rather, cognitions and behaviour and the environment must receive equal and specific attention.

Symbolic interactionism provides one such framework through which these processes may be understood.

According to symbolic interactionism (Mead 1934), the behaviours we engage in are shaped through our interaction with others. In such interactions, participants bring their own understandings and expectations of appropriate behaviours. Behaviour is then shaped by the mutual responses of the participants – a process termed 'the negotiated order'. Existing patterns of behaviour are therefore open to modification and change dependent upon the individuals involved and the circumstances they find themselves in. Central to this approach is the notion of negotiation of behaviour within a social system. In the language of social cognition theory, the behaviours we adopt are a consequence of our changing understandings of the social norms relevant to any behaviour and our own attitudes towards that behaviour. The groups with whom these relationships are negotiated, and from whom social norms are derived, differ over the lifespan. During adolescence, family and peer groups form the primary behavioural influences (Botvin and Eng 1982). During adulthood, the influence of one's own family of origin diminish. However, comparisons and behavioural negotiations with peer groups and a developing family continue throughout the life course (Backett and Davison 1995).

Many behaviours, including those related to health, arise from negotiation within the family and from individuals', sometimes shared, understandings of its needs (Graham 1985). Backett (1990), for example, found that women were less likely to exercise regularly than their male partners. These differences frequently did not correspond with desired levels of exercise. Rather, they reflected women's negotiated role within their family, and their affording higher priority to other family commitments than their own participation in regular exercise. Similarly, although a majority of women remain the main provider of food within the household, they may actually exert little control over the choice of foodstuffs. Instead, they frequently find themselves having to negotiate with a variety of differing food choices of family members – a process often involving some degree of family conflict (Kerr and Charles 1983). Backett (1990) described a process of family negotiation through which parents negotiated meals comprising both 'bad' (what the children want to eat) and 'good' (what they consider to be healthy) elements. Parents may also choose to provide healthy role models which contrast with their own behaviour of choice. This may lead to changes in parental behaviour as they adopt healthier behaviours; it frequently leads to furtive behaviour to avoid children observing smoking and poor dietary habits (Backett 1990). Transmission of behaviour is not simply a downward process. Mintel (1991), for example, reported that children between the ages of 5 and 12 act as significant influences on their parents' shopping content.

The pressures of parenthood may significantly affect the behaviours in which people engage. Under such pressure, the frequency of health-damaging behaviours may increase, particularly where material circumstances are poor and resources are low. Smoking, for example, may act as a convenient way to relieve high levels of stress and tension (Graham 1985). Alcohol consumption may increase for similar reasons, particularly among men (Westman *et al.* 1985). Parents may also be neglectful of their own health in order to protect their children at times of economic hardship, using limited resources to provide them a good diet, by sometimes doing without themselves (Backett 1990).

Responses to environmental pressure may not always be negative, however. Gottlieb and Green (1984) found exercise levels to increase among men, but not women, when facing high levels of stress. About one-fifth of women smokers, and particularly those aged below 35 years, stop smoking while pregnant, while an even greater percentage reduce their alcohol consumption to within the weekly recommended limit (Waterson and Murray-Lyon 1989). A smaller percentage of fathers also reduce their consumption of tobacco and alcohol (Waterson *et al.* 1990). Less positively, many women who stop smoking during pregnancy resume once they are no longer pregnant. Literature examining the role of women within the family and the implications of this for their own health represents a rich source of theory and data; we would direct the reader to Graham (1985) and Oakley (1974) for a comprehensive analysis.

Family pressures increase at particular times during the life cycle, for example when financial pressures exceed the family resources. Oppenheimer (1974) identified three such 'life cycle squeezes': the first when young couples attempt to set up home together, the second in middle age when supporting older children, and the third in retirement. The financial strains during these periods can often mean that one person has to work longer or a partner has to go out to part-time work. Such stresses may increase risk for disease. Arber *et al.* (1985), for example, found that full-time working mothers under the age of 40 reported many more symptoms of ill-health than part-time workers. They also found that the beneficial effects of work outside the home were dependent on social circumstances and family responsibilities. The most detrimental effects were experienced by women with no financial resources to help support their multiple roles.

This complex process of negotiations within the family, and its systemic responses to outside pressures, suggests that attempts to facilitate behavioural change may usefully address the family as a system, rather than as a series of isolated individuals. One of the few health promotion initiatives to even attempt such an approach is reported by Johnson and Nicklas (1995). Their 'Heart Smart Family' involved a systems approach to improving cardiovascular health of entire families. They argued that by involving the whole family system in change, social support and individuals' self-confidence are enhanced, and the likelihood of the adoption and maintenance of new behaviours increased. Their programme was targeted at families with children identified as at high risk for CHD. It involved a 12 to 16-week programme which minimized didactic approaches and focused on increasing awareness of health issues, skills development and problem-solving skills. Following the programme, parents evidenced lowered blood pressures, increased exercise levels, and decreased intake of total fat, saturated fat and sodium. A clinically significant reduction in children's blood pressure was also observed.

Process evaluation

A talk by Margaret Chesney (1996), President of the American Health Psychology Section, highlighted the need to develop effective health promotion programmes, and to do so quickly. In the case of just one disease process, HIV infection, she argued that effective programmes in the future could save millions of lives. Critical to the development of such programmes, she suggested, is high quality research which will allow us to better understand the processes involved in changing behaviour both at an individual and a population level and which will allow us to refine and develop our interventions to make them maximally effective. Effective research is critical to the future development of health promotion. With this in mind, the next section of this chapter addresses a number of issues concerning the evaluation of health promotion initiatives, particularly those which attempt to assess the process of change.

Research in health promotion should involve both theoretical and applied studies. The former examine and increase our understanding of the theoretical processes underpinning health promotion. The latter examine how such theories can be applied in the field. Of course, many studies combine the two elements. Here, however, we concentrate on issues pertinent to applied research: the evaluation of health promotion programmes themselves.

This type of research has proven remarkably difficult to conduct, partly as a consequence of a variety of problems facing researchers in the area. Any health gains generally follow behavioural change some years or even decades later. In addition, changes in behaviour within the general population are frequently incremental and difficult to ascribe to one particular intervention. The research methods employed by many programmes have also proved to be inappropriate, and classic experimental methods have proven difficult to implement in the 'real world' in which most health promotion initiatives and researchers are involved.

A number of researchers have offered frameworks for linking research to the development and evaluation of innovative health promotion policies or initiatives. Best *et al.* (1986), for example, identified a number of consecutive stages through which such a process should progress. In the first, the prevalence and nature of health problems or psychosocial risk indicators, such as smoking or poor housing, within the target community are determined. These data are then used to determine the intervention targets. The second stage involves the development of the intervention method. In this, small pilot experimental studies are conducted to permit comparisons of alternative intervention methods and to examine the influence of individual differences and environmental factors on outcomes. In the third stage, interventions which have proven successful in the pilot stage are implemented on a wider population and similarly evaluated. Finally (in the case of expensive and innovative interventions) demonstration or dissemination studies can be used to determine the extent to which the interventions can be conducted by other groups and in other settings. This allows an assessment of intervention implementation in the real world, through for example measuring public and professional views on intervention acceptability and identifying structural constraints to implementation.

Nutbeam *et al.* (1990) identify a further, and generally neglected type of study, in which the *process* by which any changes achieved is evaluated. This type of research helps identify relevant targets for interventions and establish effective programme approaches by increasing our understanding of the causal links between methods and end-points and how programmes are received and disseminated through the population. One example from the North Karelia heart disease prevention project (Puska *et al.* 1985) demonstrates how process evaluation may help programme development (see Chapter 7, pages 122–3). By the end of the active intervention phase in Karelia, population levels of blood pressure had fallen significantly. While this may be viewed as a successful outcome, we do not know how it was achieved. They may be consequent to behavioural changes; they may have been a result of hypertensive medication prescribed following health screening. Without this information it is difficult to judge where to put resources in future programmes.

In a useful review of process evaluation in health promotion, Dehar *et al.* (1993) suggested that process evaluation should include examination of both the process of programme development and delivery and its impact on those to whom it was addressed. Components included programme planning and the sequence of implementation, programme structure, components and delivery systems, contextual factors relevant to programme operation, participation rates and participant characteristics, levels of community awareness of programmes and resources employed for programme implementation.

While some centres of excellence report relevant data, many do not (see Nutbeam *et al.* 1990), and when process data is reported, it is frequently confined to programme participation rates or reported exposure to interventions. Even these apparently simple measures have been used inconsistently, with wide variations given to their meaning in different studies. In a review of worksite interventions, for example, Glasgow *et al.* (1993) noted that individual participation in a programme has variously been operationalized as intent to participate, registration of entry to a programme, continuous attendance, or an attempt to change behaviour. At the organizational level, participation has been measured as the reported presence of any health promotion activity, agreement to participate in a health promotion programme, and committing resources to programmes. An additional problem is that published studies may provide an inflated estimate of overall participation rates. Biases in journal editing and reviewing can lead to a higher percentage of studies reporting high participation rates being published than those which report low participation rates.

Measures of exposure to a programme provide another apparently simple measure of the ability of a programme to affect its target population. However, this information, usually gained through population surveys, typically involves retrospective self-reported experiences of exposure. These may be highly inaccurate. Underestimates may result, for example, from respondents not being aware of, or forgetting, their contact with a particular project, even if they have changed their behaviour as a consequence. Measures are also frequently unstandardized, varying from knowledge of a programme's existence to measures of the number of hours of involvement in a project or attendance at particular events or activities (Glasgow *et al.* 1993).

Participation and exposure to programme rates provide very basic process data. However, an imperative for health promotion research is to develop more sensitive measures and research methods to identify more effectively how an audience interacts with programmes. The environmental and social context in which health promotion initiatives are set necessarily impacts on their outcomes. New health promotion programmes do not interact with a naive audience, fully receptive to their messages. They encounter pre-existing social, cultural, and behavioural norms which may either inhibit or facilitate their impact. One rather dramatic example indicates how pre-existing beliefs may adversely impact on the effectiveness of a whole population health promotion programme. In the 1980s, rates of CHD in eastern European countries were high and rising. In order to reduce the incidence of disease, the Polish government established a programme exhorting the population to reduce their consumption of fatty meat and to increase consumption of vegetables, fruit, and so on. The public response was immediately to increase their consumption of fatty meat! The reason for this increase was that the call to eat less meat was thought to indicate a future meat shortage. Accordingly, many people decided to buy, and eat, as much meat as possible before this (non-existent) shortage occurred (Kazimiercz Wreszniewski, Warsaw Medical School, personal communication).

The workplace also has established cultural, social, and behavioural norms (Zimmerman and Connor 1989). Independently of any health promotion programme, these influence stress levels, motivation and barriers to behavioural change. Factors such as changes in the size and constitution of the reserve labour force, and employees' terms and conditions will affect workers' health behaviours and the outcomes of workplace programmes (Steele and Thomas 1978). The process of evaluation may also contribute to changes. Best *et al.* (1986), for example noted that when clinical treatment programmes are implemented in 'real world' contexts such as the workplace, attrition rates for participants can be four times higher than those reported in well-funded high profile research initiatives.

Understanding resistance to knowledge transmission is particularly important to health promotion, just as being able to work within such social processes is crucial to success. This complicating aspect of social life need not be seen as an obstacle to health education; it can be used to positive effect. There is a need to explore how health promotion programmes are adapted and transformed by subcultures. Most evaluations assume that behavioural change is either mostly or solely the result of outside intervention. They place emphasis on the success or failure of the communication and intervention strategy at the expense of understanding the manner in which messages and programmes are received and responded to. In contrast, ethnography and qualitative methods may be used to identify the process of understanding and transmission of health promotion messages and social contextual factors that may influence such behaviours. Examples of the utility of such research are provided by Graham (1985) and Backett (1990).

Reorienting health promotion towards positive health

The World Health Organization (1958) has stated that health is 'a state of complete physical, mental and social well-being and not merely the absence of disease or infirmity'. This statement suggests that an important role for health promotion should be to actively enhance quality of life and well-being, not simply to prevent disease. Such a development involves both adopting new strategies of working and using or developing new outcome measures to assess the impact of such initiatives.

Defining and measuring positive health

Jenkins (1992) has cogently argued that the outcome of health promotion initiatives should no longer be measured simply through measures of cognitive or behavioural change. Rather, outcome measures should include subjective feelings of well-being and functioning relevant to a number of health domains, including the biological, psychological, social and economic. Developing appropriate measures, which can be used to measure the outcome of differing intervention types, in differing settings, and attempting to change different aspects of lifestyle has proven difficult. However, a number of groups, including the World Health Organization Quality of Life Group (see Baric 1994), are involved in the development of such measures. Two forms of outcome appear most pertinent to health promotion: those of 'quality of life' and 'subjective health'. Despite the lack of appropriate measures for health promotion these constructs have been subjected to considerable research. Here we review some of the relevant literature, providing a very brief introduction into a complex area. For more detailed discussions we would direct the reader to Bowling (1995) and Stainton Rogers (1991).

Until now, the majority of well-evaluated health promotion programmes and related health surveys have been concerned with the presence or absence of risk factors for disease and of disease itself. Where psychological health has been considered, this too has been measured in terms of the presence or absence of psychological distress or psychiatric morbidity, not 'wellness' or quality of life (Dalgard *et al.* 1991). The most frequently measured constructs are those of anxiety and depression (e.g. Department of Health 1992). The General Health Questionnaire (Goldberg 1972), for example, actually measures psychiatric morbidity; scores above a specified cut-off point identify individuals likely to be given some form of psychiatric diagnosis if seen by a psychiatrist. Similarly, widely used questionnaires such as the State-Trait Anxiety Inventory and the Beck Depression Inventory (Beck *et al.* 1988) measure degrees of distress. Significantly, perhaps, an attempt to group together a series of measures for use by health professionals termed A Mental Health Portfolio (Milne 1992), identified measures under the headings of: psychological adjustment to illness, depression, anxiety, interpersonal difficulties, and so on. These categories clearly reflect an approach based on psychopathology, not positive health. A number of solutions could be offered to reorientate the focus of outcome measures used in future health promotion programmes toward positive health.

Quality of life is a multidimensional concept measuring social, mental and physical health. It has variously been described as encompassing stress coping skills, the presence of social networks, support, and social integration, life satisfaction, self-esteem, happiness and physical fitness (Lamb *et al.* 1988). Unfortunately these variables are frequently measured in isolation from each other using a wide variety of scales and with little consensus as to theoretical content (Stull 1987). Despite these problems, measures of each domain of quality of life offer areas for development in health promotion and some consensus of definition can be found. Happiness, for example, concerns an individual's affective responses to life events (usually over a recent time period), and life satisfaction involves a cognitive evaluation of achievements judged against an individual's own aspirations or the achievements of significant others (Bowling 1995). In the area of well-being, the most pertinent measure would seem to be that of self-esteem (e.g. Rosenberg 1965), involving an individual's evaluation of their own worth. There are potential difficulties in utilizing such measures in evaluation designs, not least their global nature. It would prove difficult to attribute changes (or no changes) to specific initiatives; one solution would be to use domain-specific satisfaction or happiness measures.

The influence of social health, including social networks and social support as a moderator of health status has been noted on a number of occasions throughout the book, and there is strong evidence to suggest that good social health may usefully form an outcome measure for programmes in its own right (e.g. Hersey *et al.* 1984). Definitions of social networks and social support have varied markedly (Thoits 1982). Israel and Shurman (1990) identified three domains of social support: emotional (respect and comfort), instrumental (material help) and cognitive support (information and advice), the maintenance of social identity and social outreach (access to social contacts). Vitaliano *et al.* (1985) also identified emotional and instrumental support domains in their model of coping. In contrast, Kaplan (1975) identified a much broader set of domains, including sexual satisfaction, work achievements, financial security, family support, friendships and position in the social hierarchy.

Perhaps the most common distinction between social networks and support is that the former reflects the quantity of relationships that an individual has with others, while social support refers to the quality of those relationships and type of aid provided and ease of access to them (see Bowling 1995). The distinction between the objective size of the available support system and the subjective support gained from its members is an important one. Clearly, without at least some members in a social network, high quality social support will be unavailable. However, even then it is not guaranteed. The majority of research has taken a very narrow measure of social health (see Bowling 1995), typically measuring the presence or absence of spouse or family members or the size, composition and availability of wider networks. However, there is increasing evidence that the quality of support available is the important mediator of well-being and health status (see Bowling 1995; Lazarus and Folkman 1984).

Most assessments of quality of life measure constructs, such as self-esteem or happiness, considered relevant by those developing a theory or implementing an intervention. They are top-down models, and constructs are typically measured through formal questionnaires. Lay perceptions of health, in contrast, are understandings of health held by the population of interest. They are identified through the use of informal interviews, which do not constrain the individual to predetermined responses. Instead of the theory (implicit or explicit) guiding the questions to be asked and therefore shaping the answers to fit the imposed theory, the understanding of health gained by this method is derived from the answers given to broad and unconfining questions.

One of the earliest studies of lay perceptions of health was reported by Herzlich (1973). She found that respondents conceptualized health along three dimensions. Health was variously considered as the absence of disease, a reserve to be built up and drawn upon when ill, and a state of equilibrium between the individual's physical resources, mental well-being and social relations. More recent studies have shown lay understandings of health to differ according to age, socio-economic status and gender. Blaxter (1990), for example, found that young people considered health as being an absence of 'bad habits' such as smoking and drinking, reflecting conventionally defined causes of ill-health rather than concepts of health. Young women placed emphasis on concepts of energy and vitality or a combination of the two. This included concepts such as liveliness and alertness, exemplified by not staying in bed and having good relationships with those around them such as family and friends. For men and women approaching middle age, concepts of health became much more complex and diffuse, emphasizing a more rounded state encompassing both physical and mental well-being. This included such things as being happy and relaxed and living life to the full. The idea of vitality remained, but for older men this was expressed in terms of enthusiasm for paid work and for older women ability to tackle housework. Women in particular, defined health in terms of social fulfilment, including their attitude to others and their ability to get on with others.

Definitions of positive health may not only vary by demographics but may also be determined by the social environment. Differences have been found, for example, in the types of health concepts that can be raised in the home environment (Backett 1990). Whereas women found many contexts in which to raise issues of health such as diet, exercise and preventive health behaviour, men tended to raise issues directly related to illness or to physical fitness and sports. This variety of definitions of health calls into question the use of objective scales to measure health status. However this very variety and their interdependence on socio-demographic and cultural factors makes the development of alternatives difficult. Hunt *et al.* (1986), for example, commented on the difficulty of developing a discriminating scale based on lay definitions of health during the development of the Nottingham Health Profile. However, work by O'Boyle *et al.* (see Bowling 1995) who asked individuals to list and rate the five areas they considered were most important to their quality of life suggests a fruitful way forward. The significant challenge for health promotion may be to develop more qualitative techniques that examine perceptions of health in their social context.

Positive health as a focus for health promotion

The development of measures of positive health should be accompanied by the development of health promotion interventions that focus on positive health rather than, or in addition to, the reduction of risk factors. This again reflects definitions provided by WHO (1986: 1) of health promotion as

the process of enabling people to increase control over, and to improve, their health. To reach a state of complete physical, mental and social well-being, an individual or group must be able to identify and to realize aspirations, to satisfy needs, and to change or cope with the environment . . . Therefore, health promotion is not just the responsibility of the health sector, but goes beyond healthy lifestyles to well-being.

To consider how this may be achieved, we return to the concepts of community encountered earlier. A number of definitions of community have been provided by health promotion theorists (e.g. Hawe 1994; Tonnes and Tilford 1994). On one level community has been operationalized as a 'population', in other words a large group of people (often defined by geographical location) who are the subject of large-scale interventions such as the mass media campaigns discussed in Chapter 6. Another understanding of the community is as a 'setting', that is, as a resource to support and promote healthy behaviours. This may involve the use of existing organizations and opinion leaders to transmit health messages, change perceptions of social norms and bring about environmental change, as discussed in Chapters 5 and 7. Both approaches tend to be proscriptive, viewing the community as something to be operated upon.

A third approach views the community as a 'social system', the members of which can identify their own health problems and identify strategies through which these may be remedied. This is best summed up by Ross and Lappin's (1967) definition of community development as where

a community identifies its needs or objectives, orders (or ranks) these needs or objectives, develops the confidence and will to work at these needs or objectives, finds the resources (internal and/or external) to deal with these needs and objectives [and] takes action.

Here, an ecological view of health is taken, and health promoters work with communities; their goal is to empower individuals to gain control over their lives.

In a review of community psychology and community development, Hawe (1994) suggested that they share the same conceptual roots. Sarason (1974) argued that community psychology should concern itself with the individual's need to feel a sense of belonging to those around them as an antidote to the alienation of modern life. Iscoe (1974) developed this argument further, by suggesting that community psychologists should concern themselves with building competent communities that could care for their members and use their own skills to identify problems and offer solutions. Later, Rappaport (1981) stressed the need for community psychology to focus on empowering individuals and organizations in order to help them gain control over their lives. Empowerment has frequently been defined as community participation (Tonnes and Tilford 1994). However, they are different concepts. Empowerment (through, for example, increased feelings of self-efficacy) does not necessarily lead to participation and participation does not necessarily lead to empowerment. Zimmerman (1990) argued that individuals can develop feelings of empowerment through community or organizational involvement even if the community or organization fails to achieve any desired structural change. He considered participation to be a beneficial process in itself as it can reduce feelings of hopelessness, and positively affect psychological health on measures such as social support, coping and problem-solving skills (Chesler and Chesney 1988), and personal competence (Kieffer 1984) without having to impact on the environments. However, participation without any positive outcomes may represent tokenism and over an extended period may increase feelings of hopelessness.

Recognizing that empowerment and community participation may be related but not synonymous should lead health promotion to concern itself with strategies that enhance individual feelings of belonging and life skills, and facilitate structural changes that increase group participation. With this approach, measures that have been traditionally viewed as processes therefore become important outcomes. Social measures may include changes in intra- and inter-group processes, the development of grass roots organizations, increased participation in decision-making and changes in group power relationships (such as increased financial resources and access to health care or the media). Individual measures would be of feelings of empowerment in combination with measures of personal competencies, self-esteem, self-efficacy and locus of control.

This type of approach, which places the emphasis of health promotion initiatives on personal growth, development and empowerment, shares many of the assumptions of the psychological perspective of humanism (e.g. Rogers 1951; Maslow 1970). With its roots in the early 1960s, humanism began with the founding of the Association of Humanistic Psychology which offered an alternative view of human nature to that of behaviourism and psychoanalysis. The association identified three broad principles that defined their approach, two of which have particular reference to health promotion. The first was a concern with the subjective inner world of the individual, the individual phenomenology. The investigation of this inner world required the psychologist to become a partner with the individual in the search for meaning. This may be considered analogous to the relationship between health promoters and individuals offered in community development. Second, the approach stated that the ultimate value is placed on the person; the objective of research is to understand the person, not to develop theories that could predict or control behaviour.

Finally, and most importantly in this context, was the emphasis placed on human growth and development. Rogers and his fellow humanists stated that individuals are motivated by a desire to develop and self-actualize, a tendency toward fulfilment of all capabilities. Maslow (1970) proposed a hierarchy of needs, from basic biological needs such as hunger and thirst, upwards through safety needs (security and lack of danger), to belongingness and love needs (affiliation with and acceptance by others), esteem needs (competence and approval from others), cognitive needs (to understand and explore), aesthetic needs (order and beauty) to self-actualization (to find fulfilment and realize potential). He argued that only when lower needs are satisfied could more complex psychological needs become important motivators. The emphasis here is on psychological and social aspects of health and there is a recognition that material resources and social structures either enable or hinder an individual's growth and satisfying of needs.

Although having a significant influence on therapeutic techniques (Rogers 1967; Egan 1990), humanism has largely been neglected within the design and evaluation of health promotion initiative. Taylor (1990), however, identified two possible approaches to health promotion using this perspective. The first, a humanistic approach, takes a client-centred approach, and involves the individual determining their health needs and developing the resources and skills to meet them. The second, a more radical humanist approach, again focused on client-centred participatory learning, but also recognizes that such learning occurs within a social context of relationships. According to this model, health promotion should encourage the development of social, organizational and economic networks to support individual change. This, he argued, should lead to the development of community groups and collective and individual empowerment. Evaluations of such programmes are rare. This may be due to the historical emphasis on CHD programmes and behavioural risk factors and the difficulties of measuring positive physical and mental health. Now may be the time to proceed.

Summary and conclusions

In this chapter we considered further the implications of social context on behaviour, viewing behaviour as being influenced by, and in turn influencing, the behaviour of others within the individual's social environment. We noted also that the source of such influence may change throughout the lifespan. Behaviour and health are further influenced by the economic and cultural environment in which the individual is situated. We argue, therefore, that health promotion initiatives need to take into account these moderators of behaviour and health and not simply target individuals as though isolated from such influences.

In addition, in accordance with WHO, we argue that interventions should be focused not only on reducing the incidence of disease, but also on increasing individual well-being. Finally, we suggest that those involved in health promotion should not only seek to impose initiatives arising from the philosophies and priorities of national and international bodies. Rather, they should also work to encourage communities themselves to identify health priorities and means through which these may be achieved. Such a process would ensure that health promotion works with and for individuals and communities, rather than simply imposing upon them.

Suggested reading

Backett, K.C. and Davison, C. (1995) Lifecourse and lifestyle: the social and cultural location of health behaviours. *Social Science and Medicine*, 40: 629–38.

Bloomberg, L., Meyers, J. and Braverman, M. (1994) The importance of social interaction: a new perspective on social epidemiology, social risk factors and health. *Health Education Quarterly*, 21: 447–63.

Bowling, A. (1995) *Measuring Health: A Review of Quality of Life Measurement Scales.* Buckingham: Open University Press.

Green L. and Lewis, F. (1986) *Measurement and Evaluation in Health Education and Health Promotion.* Palo Alto, CA: Mayfield Publishing Company.

Murphy, S. and Bennett, P. (1994) Psychological perspectives on young adults' health behaviour: some implications for health promotion. In G. Penny, P. Bennett and M. Herbert (eds) *Health Psychology: A Lifespan Perspective.* Reading: Harwood Academic Publishers.

Stainton Rodgers, W. (1991) *Explaining Health and Illness: An Exploration of Diversity.* Hemel Hempstead: Harvester Wheatsheaf.

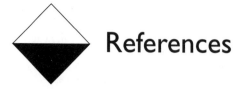 # References

Abbott, S. (1988) Talking about AIDS. Report for AIDS Action Council, Canberra. *National Bulletin*, August: 24–7.

Abraham, C.S., Sheeran, P., Abrams, D. and Spears, R. (1995) Health beliefs and teenage condom use: a prospective study. *Psychology and Health*, 11: 641–55.

Aday, L.A. (1975) Economic and non-economic barriers to the use of needed medical services. *Medical Care*, 18: 447–56.

Adler, N., Boyce, T., Chesney, M., Cohen, S., Kahn, R. and Syme, S. (1994) Socio-economic status and health: the challenge of the gradient. *American Psychologist*, 49: 15–24.

Agras, W.S., Southam, M.A. and Taylor, C.B. (1983) Long-term persistence of relaxation-induced blood pressure lowering during the working day. *Journal of Consulting and Clinical Psychology*, 51: 792–4.

Aitken, P.P., Eadie, D.R., Hastings, G.B. and Haywood, A.J. (1991) Predisposing effects of cigarette advertising on children's intentions to smoke when older. *British Journal of Addiction*, 86: 383–90.

Aitken, P.P., Leathar, D.S. and Scott, A.C. (1988) Ten to sixteen year olds' perceptions of advertisements for alcoholic drinks. *Alcohol and Alcoholism*, 23: 491–500.

Aitken, P.P., Leathar, D.S. and Squair, S.I. (1986) Children's awareness of cigarette brand sponsorship of sports and games in the UK. *Health Education Research, Theory and Practice*, 1: 203–11.

Ajzen I. (1985) From intentions to action: a theory of planned behavior. In J. Kuhl and J. Beckman (eds) *Action control: From Cognitions to Behaviors*. New York: Springer.

Ajzen I. (1991) The theory of planned behaviour. *Organizational Behavior and Human Decision Processes*, 50: 179–211.

Ajzen, I. and Fishbein, M. (1980) *Understanding Attitudes and Predicting Social Behavior.* Englewood Cliffs, NJ: Prentice-Hall.

Alexander, H.M., Callcott, R., Dobson, A.J. *et al.* (1983) Cigarette smoking and drug use in schoolchildren: IV-factors associated with changes in smoking behaviour. *International Journal of Epidemiology*, 12: 59–66.

Allard, R. (1989) Beliefs about AIDS as determinants of preventive practices and of support of coercive measures. *American Journal of Public Health*, 74: 448–52.

Ames, G.M. and Janes, C.R. (1987) Heavy and problem drinking in an American blue-collar population: implications for prevention. *Social Science and Medicine*, 25: 949–60.

Amos, A. (1992) Why children start smoking – the health education challenge. *British Journal of Addiction*, 87: 18–21.

Anderson, P., Cremona, A., Paton, A., Turner, C. and Wallace, P. (1993) The risk of alcohol. *Addiction*, 88: 1493–508.

Anderson, P. and Scott, E. (1992) The effect of general practitioners' advice to heavy drinking men. *British Journal of Addiction*, 87: 891–900.

Antonovsky, A. (1987) *Unravelling the Mystery of Health: How People Manage Stress and Stay Well*. San Francisco, CA: Jossey-Bass.

Apsler, R. and Sears, D. (1968) Warnings, personal involvement, and attitude change. *Journal of Personality and Social Psychology*, 9: 162–6.

Arber, S. (1989) Gender and class inequalities in health: Understanding the differentials. In J. Fox (ed.) *Health Inequalities in European Countries*. Aldershot: Gower Publishing Company.

Arber, S., Gilbert, G. and Dale, A. (1985) Paid employment and women's health: a benefit or a source of role strain? *Sociology of Health and Illness*, 7: 375–400.

Asch, P. and Levy, D.T. (1987) Does the minimum drinking age affect traffic fatalities? *Journal of Policy Analysis and Management*, 6: 180–92.

Ashton, H. and Stepney, R. (1982) *Smoking: Psychology and Pharmacology*. London: Tavistock Publications.

Ashton, J. (1992) *Healthy Cities*. Buckingham: Open University Press.

Atkin, C., Hocking, J. and Block, M. (1984) Teenage drinking . . . does advertising make a difference? *Journal of Communications*, 34: 157–67.

Austoker, J. (1994) Diet and cancer. *British Medical Journal*, 308: 1610–14.

Bachman, J.G., Johnson, L.D., O'Malley, P.M. and Humphrey, H. (1988) Explaining the recent decline in marijuana use: differentiating the effects of perceived risks, disapproval, and general life-style factors. *Journal of Health and Social Behaviour*, 29: 92–112.

Backett, K. (1990) Studying health in families: A qualitative approach. In A. Cunningham, S. Burly and N. McKeganey (eds) *Readings in Medical Sociology*. London: Routledge.

Backett, K.C. and Davison, C. (1995) Lifecourse and lifestyle: the social and cultural location of health behaviours. *Social Science and Medicine*, 40: 629–38.

Bagozzi, R.P. and Warshaw, P.R. (1990) Trying to consume. *Journal of Consumer Research*, 17: 127–40.

Balarajan, R. and Raleigh, V. (1993) *Ethnicity and Health in England*. London: HMSO.

Balarajan, R. and Yuen, P. (1986) British smoking and drinking habits: variations by country of birth. *Community Medicine*, 8: 237–9.

Bandura, A. (1969) *Principles of Behavior Modification*. New York: Holt, Rhinehart & Winston.

Bandura, A. (1977) Self-efficacy: toward a unifying theory of behavioural change. *Psychological Review*, 84: 191–215.

Bandura, A. (1986) *Social Foundations of Thought and Action: A Social Cognitive Theory*. Englewood Cliffs, NJ: Prentice-Hall.

Barefoot, J.C., Dahlstrom, J.W. and Williams, R.B. (1983) Hostility, CHD incidence and total mortality: a 25-year follow-up study of 225 physicians. *Psychosomatic Medicine*, 45: 59–63.

Baric, L. (1994) *Health Promotion and Health Education in Practice: The Organisational model*. Hale Barns: Barns Publications.

Barker, R.M. and Baker, M.R. (1990) Incidence of cancer in Bradford Asians. *Journal of Epidemiology and Community Health*, 44: 125–9.

Barton, J., Chassin, L., Presson, C.C. and Sherman, S.J. (1982) Social image factors as motivators of smoking initiation in early and middle adolescence. *Child Development*, 53: 1499–511.

Baumgardner, M.H., Leippe, M.R., Ronis, D.L. and Greenwald, A.G. (1983) In search of reliable persuasion effects: associative interference and persistence of persuasion in a message-dense environment. *Journal of Personality and Social Psychology*, 45: 524–37.

Beck, A.T. (1976) *Cognitive Therapy and the Emotional Disorders*. New York: International Universities Press.

Beck, A.T., Steer, R.A. and Garbin, M.G. (1988) Psychometric properties of the Beck Depression Inventory: twenty five years of evaluation. *Clinical Psychology Review*, 8: 77–100.

Becker, M.H. (1974) The health belief model and personal health behavior. *Health Education Monographs*, 2: 324–508.

Becker, M.H., Haefner, D.P. and Maiman, L.A. (1977) The health belief model in the prediction of dietary compliance: a field experiment. *Journal of Health and Social Behavior*, 18: 348–66.

Bellingham, K. and Gillies, P. (1993) Evaluation of an AIDS education programme for young adults. *Journal of Epidemiology and Community Health*, 47: 134–8.

Bendick, M. and Cantu, M.C. (1978) The literacy of welfare clients. *Social Services Review*, March: 56–68.

Bennett, P. (1993) *Counselling for Heart Disease*. Leicester: British Psychological Society.

Bennett, P. (1994) Should we modify Type A behaviour in patients with manifest coronary heart disease? *Behavioural and Cognitive Psychotherapy*, 22: 125–45.

Bennett, P. (1995) Disorders of the gut. In A. Broome and S. Llewelyn (eds) *Health Psychology: Processes and Applications*. (2nd edn) London: Chapman and Hall.

Bennett, P. and Carroll, D. (1997) Stress management approaches to the prevention of heart disease. In S. Palmer and W. Dryden (eds) *Stress Management and Counselling: Theory, Practice, Research and Methodology*. Cassell: London.

Bennett, P., Moore, L., Smith, A., Murphy, S. and Smith, C. (1995) Health locus of control and value for health as predictors of dietary behaviour. *Psychology and Health*, 10: 41–54.

Bennett, P., Norman, P., Murphy, S., Moore, L. and Tudor-Smith, C. (1997) Health locus of control and value for health in smokers and non-smokers. *Health Psychology*, 16: 179–82.

Bennett, P. and Rowe, A. (in press) Adherence to asthma preventive drug regimes: a test of protection motivation theory. *British Journal of Health Psychology*.

Bennett, P. and Smith, C. (1992) Parents' attitudinal and social influences on childhood vaccination. *Health Education Research, Theory and Practice*, 7: 341–8.

Bennett, P., Smith, C. and Nugent, Z. (1991a) Patterns of drinking in Wales. *Alcohol and Alcoholism*, 26: 367–74.

Bennett, P., Smith, C., Nugent, Z. and Panter, C. (1991b) 'Pssst . . . the really useful guide to alcohol': evaluation of an alcohol education television series. *Health Education Research, Theory and Practice*, 6: 57–64.

Bennett, P., Wallace, L., Carroll, D. and Smith, N. (1991c) Treating Type A behaviours and mild hypertension in middle-aged men. *Journal of Psychosomatic Research*, 35: 209–23.

Bertera, R.L. (1990) Planning and implementing health promotion in the workplace: a case study of the Du Pont company experience. *Health Education Quarterly*, 17: 307–27.

Best, J.A., Cameron, R. and Grant, M. (1986) Health behaviour and health promotion. *American Journal of Health Promotion*, Fall: 48–56.

Bettinghaus, E. (1986) Health promotion and the knowledge attitude behaviour continuum. *Preventive Medicine*, 15: 475–91.

Black, D.R. and Smith, M.A. (1994) Reducing alcohol consumption among university students: recruitment and program design strategies based on Social Marketing Theory. *Health Education Research*, 9(3): 375–84.

Blair, S.N., Piserchia, P.V., Wilbur, C.S. and Crowder, J.H. (1986) A public health intervention model for work-site health promotion. Impact on exercise and physical fitness in a health promotion plan after 24 months. *Journal of the American Medical Association*, 255: 921–6.

Blakey, V. and Frankland, J. (1995) Evaluating HIV prevention for women prostitutes in Cardiff. *Health Education Journal*, 54: 131–42.

Blane, D. (1985) An assessment of the Black Report's explanations of health inequalities. *Sociology of Health and Illness*, 7: 423–45.

Blane, T. and Hewitt, L. (1977) Alcohol and youth: an analysis of the literature. Washington, National Technical Information Service, U.S. Department of Commerce.

Blaxter, M. (1983) The causes of disease: women talking. *Social Science and Medicine*, 17: 59–64.

Blaxter M. (1990) *Health and lifestyles*. London: Heinemann.

Blaxter, M. and Paterson, E. (1982) *Mothers and Daughters: A Three Generational Study of Health Attitudes and Behaviours*. London: Heinemann.

Boer, H. and Seydel, E.R. (1996) Protection motivation theory. In M. Conner and P. Norman (eds) *Predicting Health Behaviour*. Buckingham: Open University Press.

Botvin, G.J. and Eng, A. (1982) The efficiency of a multicomponent approach to the prevention of cigarette smoking. *Preventative Medicine*, 11: 199–211.

Bowling, A. (1995) *Measuring Health: A Review of Quality of Life Measurement Scales*. Buckingham: Open University Press.

Bradley, C.B. and Kegeles, S.M. (1987) The use of diabetics-specific perceived control and health belief measures to predict treatment choice and efficacy in a feasibility study of continuous subcutaneous insulin infusion pumps. *Psychology and Health*, 1: 133–46.

Bragg, B. and Marr, J. (1991) *Sexuality*. London: BMG Music Publishing Limited.

Brehm, S. and Brehm, J. (1981) *Psychological Reactance: A Theory of Freedom and Control*. New York: Academic Press.

Bremble, A., Bennett, P. and Morgan, M. (1991) Explaining health behaviours: a pilot study. Unpublished manuscript, University of Wales, Cardiff.

Breslow, L. and Enstrom, J.E. (1980) Persistence of health habits and their relationship to mortality. *Preventive Medicine*, 9: 469–83.

Brook, S. and Smith, C. (1991) Do combined oral contraceptive users know how to take their pill correctly? *The British Journal of Family Planning*, 17: 18–20.

Brotherston, J. (1976) Inequality: is it inevitable? In C.O. Carter and J. Peel (eds) *Equalities and Inequalities in Health*. London: Academic Press.

Brown, C. (1984) *Black and White Britain: The Third PSI Survey*. London: Heinemann.

Brownell, K.D. and Felix, M.R. (1987) Competitions to facilitate health promotions: review and conceptual analysis. *American Journal of Health Promotion*, 2: 28–36.

Brownson, R., Koffman, D., Novotny, T., Hughes, R. and Eriksen, M. (1995) Environmental and policy interventions to control tobacco use and prevent cardiovascular disease. *Health Education Quarterly*, 22(4): 478–98.

Buchanan, D.R., Reddy, S. and Hossain Z. (1994) Social marketing: a critical appraisal. *Health Promotion International*, 9(1): 49–57.

Bunton, R. (1992) Health promotion as social policy. In R. Bunton and G. MacDonald (eds) *Health Promotion Disciplines and Diversity*. London: Routledge.

Bunton, R. and MacDonald, G. (1992) Health promotion: discipline or disciplines? In R. Bunton and G. MacDonald (eds) *Health Promotion: Disciplines and Diversity*. London: Routledge.

Bunton, R., Murphy, S. and Bennett, P. (1991) Theories of behavioural change and their use in health promotion: some neglected areas. *Health Education Research, Theory and Practice* (special issue on theory), 6: 153–64.

Burr, M., Gilbert, J. and Holliday, R. (1989) Effects of ion changes in fat, fish, and fibre intakes on death and myocardial infarction: diet and reinfarction trial. *Lancet*, ii: 757–61.

Buttrose, I. (1987) Editorial. *AIDS and Women*, August: 34–5.

Byrne, D. (1961) The repression–sensitization scale: rationale, reliability and validity. *Journal of Personality*, 29: 344–9.

Calman, K.C. (1991) *On the State of the Public Health: The Annual Report of the Chief Medical Officer of the Department of Health for the Year 1991*. London: HMSO.

Calnan, M. (1989) Control over health and patterns of health-related behaviour. *Social Science and Medicine*, 29: 131–6.

Cameron, T. (1978) *The Impact of Drinking–Driving Countermeasures: A Review and Evaluation*. Berkeley, CA: Social Research Group Working Paper F–81.

Caplan, R. (1993) The importance of social theory for health promotion: from description to reflexivity. *Health Promotion International*, 8: 147–57.

Carleton, R.A., Lasater, T.M., Assaf, A.R., Feldman, H.A., McKinlay, S. and the Pawtucket Program Writing Group (1995) The Pawtucket Heart Health Program: community changes in cardiovascular risk factors and projected disease risk. *American Journal of Public Health*, 85: 777–85.

Carli, L.L. (1990) Gender, language, and influence. *Journal of Personality and Social Psychology*, 59: 941–51.

Carroll, D., Bennett, P. and Davey Smith, G. (1993) Health and social and material circumstances: their origins and implications. *Psychology and Health*, 8: 295–316.

Carroll, D., Davey Smith, G. and Bennett, P. (1996) Social class and health: the widening gap. *Journal of Health Psychology*, 1: 23–39.

Carstairs, V. (1970) *Channels of Communication*. Edinburgh: Scottish Home and Health Department.

Carter, S. and Carter, D. (1993) Gender differentiated receptivity to sexual education curricula by adolescents. *Health Education Research, Theory and Practice*, 8: 233–43.

Case, R.B., Heller, S.S., Case, N.B. and Moss, A.J. and the Multicenter Post-Infarction Research Group (1985) Type A behaviour and survival after acute myocardial infarction. *New England Journal of Medicine*, 312: 737–41.

Cataldo, M.F. and Coates, T.J. (1986) *Health and Industry: A Behavioral Medicine Perspective.* New York: Wiley.

Catchpole, M. (1992) *Sexually Transmitted Diseases in England and Wales 1982–1990. Community Diseases Review R1–R6.* London: Public Health Laboratories.

Central Statistics Office (1980) A change in revenue from an indirect tax change. *Economic Trends*, March: 97–107.

Chaffe, S.H. and Mutz, D.C. (1988) Comparing mediated and interpersonal communication data. In R. Hawkins, J. Wiemann and S. Pingree (eds) *Advancing Communication Science: Merging Mass and Interpersonal Processes.* Newbury Park, CA: Sage.

Chapman, S. and Fitzgerald, B. (1982) Brand preferences and advertising recall in adolescent smokers: some implications for health promotion. *American Journal of Public Health*, 72: 491–4.

Chapman, S. and Hodgson, J. (1988) Showers in raincoats. Attitudinal barriers to condom use in high risk heterosexuals. *Community Health Studies*, 12: 97–105.

Charlton, A. (1988) Evaluation of a family linked smoking programme in primary schools. *Health Education Journal*, 45: 140–4.

Chesler, M. and Chesney, B. (1988) Self-help groups: empowerment attitudes and behaviors of disabled or chronically ill persons. In H.E. Yuker (ed.) *Attitudes Toward Persons with Disabilities.* New York: Springer.

Chesney, M.A., Black, G.W., Swan, G.E. and Ward, M.M. (1987) Relaxation training at the worksite: the untreated mild hypertensive. *Psychosomatic Medicine*, 49: 250–73.

Chesney, M.A., Hecker, M.H.L. and Black, G.W. (1988) Coronary-prone components of the Type A behavior pattern in the WCGS: a new methodology. In B.K. Houston and C.R. Snyder (eds) *The Type A Behavior Pattern. Research, Theory and Intervention.* New York: Wiley.

Choukron, J.M., Raven, I. and Wagner, C. (1985) *The relationship between increases in Minimum Purchase Age for Alcoholic Beverages and the Number of Traffic Fatalities*, PA S3 – paper 85–04. Philadelphia, PA: Social Systems Department, University of Pennsylvania.

Christenson, G.M. and Kiefhaber, A. (1988) The national survey of worksite health promotion activities. *American Association of Occupational Health Nurses*, 35: 262–5.

Cinciriprini, P.M., Lapitsky, L.G., Wallfisch, A. and Mace, R. (1994) An evaluation of a multicomponent treatment program involving scheduled smoking and relapse prevention procedures: initial findings. *Addictive Behaviors*, 19: 13–22.

Cirksena, M.K. and Flora, J.A. (1995) Audience segmentation in worksite health promotion: a procedure using social marketing concepts. *Health Education Research*, 10: 211–24.

Clarke, M., Ahmed, N., Romaniuk, H., Marjot, D.H. and Murray-Lyon, I.M. (1990) Ethnic differences in the consequences of alcohol misuse. *Alcohol and Alcoholism*, 25: 9–11.

Coates, T.J. (1990) Strategies for modifying sexual behaviour for primary and secondary prevention of HIV disease. *Journal of Consulting and Clinical Psychology*, 58: 57–69.

Cochrane, R. and Bal, S.S. (1989) Mental hospital admission rates of immigrants to England: a comparison of 1971 and 1981. *Social Psychiatry and Psychiatric Epidemiology*, 24: 2–11.

Cohen, F. (1979) Personality, stress, and the development of physical illness. In G.C. Stone, F. Cohen and N.E. Adler (eds) *Health Psychology*. San Francisco, CA: Jossey-Bass.

Cohen, S. (1988) Psychosocial models of the role of social support in the etiology of physical disease. *Health Psychology*, 7: 269–97.

Cohen, S., Tyrell, D.A. and Smith, A.P. (1991) Psychological stress in humans and susceptibility to the common cold. *New England Journal of Medicine*, 325: 606–12.

Cole, R. and Holland, S. (1980) Recall of health education display materials. *Health Education Journal*, 39: 74–9.

Collins, R., Peto, R., MacMahon, S., Hebert, P., Fiebach, N.H. and Eberlain, K. (1990) Blood pressure, stroke, and coronary heart disease. Part 2. Short-term reductions in blood pressure: overview of randomised drug trials in the epidemiological context. *Lancet*, 335: 827–38.

COMMIT Research Group (1995) Community intervention trial for smoking cessation (COMMIT): II. Changes in adult cigarette smoking prevalence. *American Journal of Public Health*, 85(2): 193–200.

Conner, M. and Norman, P. (eds) (1996) *Predicting Health Behaviour: Research and Practice with Social Cognition Models*. Buckingham: Open University Press.

Conner, M., Povey, R., Bell, R. and Norman, P. (1994) 'GP intervention to produce dietary change.' Paper presented at the British Psychological Society Special Group in Health Psychology Annual Conference, Sheffield.

Cox, H. and Smith, R. (1984) Political approaches to smoking control: a comparative analysis. *Applied Economics*, 16: 569–82.

Crawford, R. (1977) You are dangerous to your health: the ideology and politics of victim blaming. *International Journal of Health Services*, 10: 365–88.

Cronkite, R.C. and Moos, R.H. (1984) The role of predisposing and moderating factors in the stress–illness relationship. *Journal of Health and Social Behavior*, 25: 372–93.

Cubis, J, Lewis, T. and Raphael, B. (1985) Correlates of pregnancy and sexual experience in Australian adolescents. *Journal of Obstetrics and Gynaecology*, 4: 237–54.

Cullen, I. (1979) Urban social policy and problems of family life: the use of an extended diary method to inform decision analysis. In C. Harris (ed.) *The Sociology of the Family: New Directions in Britain. Sociological Review Monograph 28*. Keele: University of Keele.

Cummings, K., Pechacek, T. and Shopland, D. (1994) The illegal sale of cigarettes to US minors: estimates by state. *American Journal of Public Health*, 84: 300–2.

Curtice, R. (1991) European healthy cities research – where is it? *Critical Public Health*, 1: 42–8.

Cyster, R. (1986) Setting limits. *Nursing Times*. May 7: 51–2.

Cyster, R. and McEwen, J. (1987) Alcohol education at the workplace. *Health Education Journal*, 46, 4: 156–62.

Cyster, R. and McEwen, J. (1988) Alcohol problems at work: a new approach? *Public Health*, 102: 373–9.

Dalgard, O., Sorensen, T. and Bjork, S. (1991) Community psychiatry and health promotion research. In B. Bandura and I. Kickbusch (eds) *Health Promotion Research: Towards a New Social Epidemiology*. Copenhagen: WHO.

Davey Smith, G. and Pekkanen, J. (1992) Should there be a moratorium on the use of cholesterol lowering drugs? *British Medical Journal*, 304: 431–4.

Davey Smith, G., Song, F. and Sheldon, T.A. (1993) Cholesterol lowering and mortality: the importance of considering initial level of risk. *British Medical Journal*, 306: 1367–73.

Davidson, C., Davey Smith, G. and Frankel, S. (1991) Lay epidemiology and the prevention paradox: the implications of coronary candidacy for health education. *Sociology of Health and Illness*, 13: 1–19.

Day, N.E. (1996) *The Incidence and Prevalence of AIDS and Prevalence of Other Severe HIV Diseases in England and Wales for 1995–1999*. London: PHLS Communicable Disease Report.

DeBono, K.G. and Telesca, C. (1990) The influence of source physical attractiveness on advertising effectiveness: a functional perspective. *Journal of Applied Social Psychology*, 20: 1383–95.

Decker, B.D. and Evans, R.G. (1989) Efficacy of a minimal contact version of a multimodal smoking cessation program. *Addictive Behaviors*, 14: 487–91.

DeFoe, J.R. and Breed, W. (1988/9) Consulting to change media contents: two cases in alcohol education. *International Quarterly of Community Health Education*, 4: 257–72.

DeFoe, J., Breed, W. and Breed L. (1983) Drinking on television: a five-year study. *Journal of Drug Education*, 13: 25–8.

Dehar, M.A., Casswell, S. and Duignan, P. (1993) Formative and process evaluation of health promotion and disease prevention programmes. *Evaluation Review*, 17: 204–20.

Dembroski, T., Lasater, T. and Ramirez, A. (1978) Communicator similarity, fear arousing communication and compliance with health care recommendations. *Journal of Applied Social Psychology*, 8: 254–69.

Dembroski, T.M., MacDougall, J.M., Costa, P.T. and Grandits, G.A. (1989) Components of hostility as predictors of sudden death and myocardial infarction in the Multiple Risk Factor Intervention Trial. *Psychosomatic Medicine*, 51: 514–22.

Dennehey, E., Edwards, C. and Keller, R. (1995) AIDS education intervention utilising a person with AIDS: examination and clarification. *AIDS Education and Prevention*, 7: 124–33.

Department of Health (1992) *The Health of the Nation*. London: HMSO.

Department of Health (1995) *Sensible Drinking. The Report of an interdepartmental working group*. Wetherby: Department of Health.

DiClemente, J., Zorn, J. and Temoshok, L. (1987) The association between gender, ethnicity and length of residence in the Bay Area to adolescents' knowledge and attitudes about AIDS. *Journal of Social Psychology*, 17: 216–30.

DiFranza, J.R., Richards, J.W., Paulman, P.M., Wolf-Gillespie, N., Fletcher, C., Jaffe, R.D. and Murray, D. (1991) RJR Nabisco's cartoon camel promotes camel cigarettes to children. *Journal of the American Medical Association*, 226: 3149–53.

Directorate of the Welsh Heart Programme (1986) *Heart of Wales: Clinical Results of the Welsh Heart Survey. Heartbeat Report No. 20*. Cardiff: Heartbeat Wales.

Dishman, R.K. (1982) Compliance/adherence in health-related exercise. *Health Psychology*, 1: 237–67.

Doll, J. and Orth, B. (1993) The Fishbein and Ajzen theory of reasoned action applied to contraceptive behavior: model variants and meaningfulness. *Journal of Applied Social Psychology*, 23: 395–415.

Dorn, N. (1983) *Alcohol, Youth and the State*. London: Croom Helm.

Douglas, J. (1995) Developing anti-racist health promotion strategies. In R. Burrows and S. Nettleton (eds) *The Sociology of Health Promotion*. London: Routledge.

Douglas, M. (1986) *Risk Acceptability According to the Social Sciences*. London: Routledge.

Doyle, Y. (1991) A survey of the cervical screening service in a London district, including reasons for non-attendance, ethnic responses and views on the quality of the service. *Social Science and Medicine*, 32: 953–7.

Duffy, J.C. (1981) The influence of prices, consumer incomes and advertising upon the demand for alcoholic drink in the United Kingdom: an economic study. *British Journal of Alcohol and Alcoholism*, 16: 200–8.

Duffy, M. (1991) Advertising and the consumption of tobacco and alcoholic drinks: a system-wide analysis. *Scottish Journal of Political Economy*, 38: 369–85.

Duhl, L.J. (1986) The Healthy City: its function and its future. *Health Promotion International*, 1: 55–60.

Dzewaltowski, D.A., Noble, J.M. and Shaw, J.M. (1990) Physical activity participation: social cognitive theory versus the theories of reasoned action and planned behavior. *Journal of Sport and Exercise Psychology*, 12: 388–405.

Egan, G. (1990) *The Skilled Helper. Models, Skills, and Methods for Effective Helping*. Monterey, CA: Brooks Cole.

Elmer, P.J., Grimm, R., Laing, B., Grandits, G., Svendsen, M., van Heel, N., Betz, E., Raines, J., Link, M., Stamler, J. and Neaton, J. (1995) Lifestyle intervention: results of the treatment of mild hypertension study (TOMHS). *Preventive Medicine*, 24: 378–88.

Eperlein, T. (1985) *The Use of Sobriety as a Deterrent: An Impact Assessment*. Phoenix, AZ: State of Arizona Statistical Analysis Center.

Erfurt, J.C., Foote, A., Heirich, M.A. and Gregg, W. (1990) Improving participation in worksite wellness programs: comparing health education classes, a menu approach, and follow-up counselling. *American Journal of Health Promotion*, 4: 270–8.

Eriksen, M.P. (1986) Workplace smoking control: rationale and approaches. *Advances in Health Education and Promotion*, 1(A): 65–103.

Everly, G.S. and Feldman, R.H.L. (1985) *Occupational Health Promotion: Health Behavior in the Worksite*. New York: Wiley.

Fagerstrom, K.O. (1982) A comparison of psychological and pharmacological treatments on smoking cessation. *Journal of Behavioral Medicine*, 5: 343–51.

Family Heart Study Group (1994) Randomised controlled trial evaluating cardiovascular screening and intervention in general practice: principal results of British family heart study. *British Medical Journal*, 308: 313–20.

Farquhar, J.W., Fortmann, S.P., Flora, J.A., Taylor, C.B., Haskell, W.L., Williams, P.T., Maccoby, N. and Wood, P.D. (1990) Effects of community-wide education on cardiovascular disease risk factors. The Stanford Five-City Project. *Journal of the American Medical Association*, 264: 359–65.

Farquhar, J.W., Maccoby, N., Wood, P.D., Alexander, J.K., Breitrose, H., Brown Jr., B.W., Haskell, W.L., McAlister, A.L., Meyer, A.J., Nash, J.D. and Stern, M.P. (1977) Community education for cardiovascular health. *Lancet*, 1: 1192–8.

Fazio, R. and Zanna, M. (1981) Direct experience and attitude behavior consistency. In L. Berkowitz (ed.) *Advances in Experimental Social Psychology. 14*. Orlando, FL: Academic Press.

Festinger, L. (1957) *A Theory of Cognitive Dissonance*. Stanford, CA: Stanford University Press.

Fielding, J. (1982) Effectiveness of Employee Health Improvement Programs. *Journal of Occupational Medicine*, 24: 907–16.

Fielding, J.E., Mason, T., Knight, K., Klesges, R. and Pelletier, K.R. (1995) A randomized trial of the IMPACT worksite cholesterol reduction program. *American Journal of Preventive Medicine*, 11: 120–3.

Fishbein, M. and Ajzen, I. (1975) *Belief, Attitude, Intention, and Behavior: An Introduction to Theory and Research*. Reading, MA: Addison-Wesley.

Flay, B.R. (1987) Mass media and smoking cessation: a critical review. *American Journal of Public Health*, 77: 153–60.

Flesch, R. (1948) A new readability yardstick. *Journal of Applied Psychology*, 32: 221–33.

Flora, J. and Maibach, E. (1990) Cognitive responses to AIDS information. The effect of issue involvement and message appeal. *Communication Research*, 17: 759–74.

Flora, J. and Thorensen, C. (1988) Reducing the risk of AIDS in adolescents. *American Psychologist*, 43: 965–70.

Foerster, S.B., Bal, D.G., Kizer, K.W., Krieg, B.F., DiSogra, L.K. and Bunch, K.L. (1995) California's 5 a day for better health campaign. An innovative population based effort to effect large scale dietary change. *American Journal of Preventive Medicine*, 11: 124–31.

Fortmann, S., Barr Taylor, C., Flora, J. and Winkleby, M. (1993) Effects of community health education on plasma cholesterol levels and diet: The Stanford Five-City Project. *American Journal of Epidemiology*, 137: 1039–55.

Fox, K.M. and Shapiro, L.M. (1988) Heart disease in Asians in Britain: commoner than in Europeans, but why? *British Medical Journal*, 297: 311–12.

Frankenhauser, M. (1979) Psychoneuroendocrine approaches to the study of emotions related to stress and coping. In D. Howe (ed.) *Nebraska Symposium on Motivation*. Lincoln, NB: University of Nebraska Press.

Franzkowiak, P. (1987) Risk taking and adolescent development. *Health Promotion*, 2: 51–60.

Freud, S. (1900/1967) *On the Interpretation of Dreams*. Harmondsworth: Penguin.

Friedman, H.L. (1989) The health of adolescents: beliefs and behaviour. *Social Science and Medicine*, 29(3): 309–15.

Friedman, M., Thoresen, C.E., Gill, J.J., Ulmer, D., Powell, L.H., Price, V.A., Brown, B., Thompson, L., Rabin, D.D., Breall, W.S., Bourg, E., Levy, R. and Dixon, T. (1986) Alteration of Type A behavior and its effect on cardiac recurrences in post-myocardial infarction patients: summary results of the Recurrent Coronary Prevention Project. *American Heart Journal*, 112: 653–65.

Fries, J.F., Fries, S.T., Parcell, C.L. and Harrington, H. (1992) Health risk changes with a low-cost individualized health promotion program: effects at up to 30 months. *American Journal of Health Promotion*, 6: 364–71.

Friestad, M. and Thorson, E. (1965) 'The role of emotion in memory for television commercials.' Paper presented at the annual meeting of the International Communication Association, Honolulu, Hawaii, June.

Fritzen, R. and Mazer, G. (1975) Effects of fear appeal and communication upon attitudes toward alcohol consumption. *Journal of Drug Education*, 5: 171–81.

Gatherer, A., Parfit, J., Porter, E. and Vessey, M. (1979) Is health education effective? *Health Education Council Monograph 2*. London: Health Education Council.

Glanz, K., Lankenau, B., Foerster, S., Temple, S., Mullis, R. and Schmid, T. (1995) Environmental and policy approaches to cardiovascular disease prevention through nutrition: opportunities for state and local action. *Health Education Quarterly*, 22: 512–27.

Glanz, K. and Rudd, J. (1990) Readability and content analysis of printed cholesterol education materials. *Patient Education and Counselling*, 16: 109–18.

Glasgow, R.E., Klesges, R.C., Mizes, J.S. and Pechacek, T.F. (1985) Quitting smoking: strategies used and variables associated with success in a stop-smoking contest. *Journal of Consulting and Clinical Psychology*, 53: 905–13.

Glasgow, R.E., McCaul, K.D. and Fisher, K.J. (1993) Participation in worksite health promotion: a critique of the literature and recommendations for future practice. *Health Education Quarterly*, 20: 391–408.

Glasgow, R.E., Terborg, J.R., Hollis, J.F., Severson, H.H. and Boles, S.M. (1995) Take heart: results from the initial phase of a work-site wellness program. *American Journal of Public Health*, 85: 209–16.

Goddard, E. and Ikin, C. (1988) *Smoking Among Secondary School Children in 1986*. London: HMSO.

Godding, P.R. and Glasgow, R.E. (1985) Self-efficacy and outcome expectations as predictors of controlled smoking status. *Cognitive Therapy and Research*, 9: 583–90.

Godfrey, C. (1990) Modelling demand. In A. Maynard and P. Tether (eds) *Preventing Alcohol and Tobacco Problems. 1.* Avebury: Economic and Social Science Research Council.

Goldberg, D. (1972) *Detection of Psychiatric Illness by Questionnaire*. Oxford: Oxford University Press.

Goldberg, E. and Comstock, G. (1980) Epidemiology of life events: frequency in general populations. *American Journal of Epidemiology*, 111: 736–52.

Gollwitzer, P.M. (1993) Goal achievement: the role of intentions. In W. Stroebe and M. Hewstone (eds) *European Review of Social Psychology, Volume 4*. Chichester: Wiley.

Gomel, N., Oldenburg, B., Simpson, J.M. and Owen, N. (1993) Work-site cardiovascular risk reduction: a randomized trial of health risk assessment, education, counseling, and incentives. *American Journal of Public Health*, 83: 1231–8.

Goodman, R.M., Wheeler, F.C. and Lee, P.R. (1995) Evaluation of the Heart to Heart Project: lessons from a community-based chronic disease prevention project. *American Journal of Health Promotion*, 9: 443–55.

Gottlieb, N. and Green, L. (1987) Ethnicity and lifestyle health risk: some possible mechanisms. *American Journal of Health Promotion*, 1: 37–45.

Gourlay, S.G., Forbes, A., Marriner, T., Pethica, D. and McNeil, J.J. (1995) Double blind trial of repeated treatment with transdermal nicotine for relapsed smokers. *British Medical Journal*, 311: 363–6.

Graham, H. (1976) Smoking in pregnancy: the attitudes of expectant mothers. *Social Science and Medicine*, 10: 399–405.

Graham, H. (1985) *Women, Health and Families*. Brighton: Harvester Press.

Green, E., Hebron, S. and Woodward, D. (1986) *Leisure and Gender. A Study of Sheffield Women's Experiences*. Report to the Economic and Social Science Research Council/Sports Council Joint Panel on Leisure Research, London.

Green, L.W. and Iverson, D.C. (1982) School health education. *Annual Review of Public Health*, 3: 321–38.

Greenfield, S., Kaplan, S. and Ware, Jr., H.J.E. (1985) Expanding patient involvement in care: effects on patient outcomes. *Annals of Internal Medicine*, 102: 520–8.

Greenland, P., Hildreth, N.G. and Maiman, L.A. (1992) Attendance pattern and characteristics of participants in public cholesterol screening. *American Journal of Preventive Medicine*, 8(3): 159–64.

Greig, R. and Raphael, B. (1989) AIDS prevention and adolescents. *Community Health Studies*, 13: 211–19.

Gruder, C.L., Cook, T.D., Hennigan, K.M., Flay, B.R., Alessis, C. and Halamaj, J. (1978) Empirical tests of the absolute sleeper effect predicted from the discounting cue hypothesis. *Journal of Personality and Social Psychology*, 36: 1061–74.

Gudykunst, W., Yoon, Y. and Nishda, T. (1987) The influence of individualism–collectivism on perceptions of communication in ingroup and outgroup relationships. *Communication Monographs*, 54: 295–306.

Haan, M.N. and Kaplan, G. (1986) The contribution of socio-economic position to minority health. In *Report of the Secretary's Task Force on Black and Minority Health*, volume 2. Washington DC: US Department of Health and Human Services.

Hall, S.M., Tunstall, C., Rugg, D., Jones, R.T. and Benowitz, N. (1985) Nicotine gum and behavioral treatment in smoking cessation. *Journal of Consulting and Clinical Psychology*, 53: 256–8.

Hall, S.M., Tunstall, C., Rugg, D., Jones, R.T. and Benowitz, N. (1987) Nicotine gum and behavioural treatment: A placebo controlled trial. *Journal of Consulting and Clinical Psychology*, 55: 603–5.

Hamburg, D.A., Elliott, G.R. and Parron, D.L. (1982) *Health and Behavior: Frontiers of Research in the Biobehavioral Sciences*. Washington DC: National Academy Press.

Hamilton, J.L. (1972) The demand for cigarettes: advertising, the health scare and the cigarette advertising ban. *Review of Economics and Statistics*, 56: 401–11.

Hancock, T. (1993) The evolution, impact and significance of the healthy cities/healthy communities movement. *Journal of Public Health Policy*, 14: 5–18.

Hansen, A. (1986) The portrayal of alcohol on television. *Health Education Journal*, 45: 127–31.

Hansen, W.B., Graham, J.W., Sobel, J.L., Shelton, D.R., Flay, B.R. and Johnson, C.A. (1987) The consistency of peer and parental influences on tobacco, alcohol, and marijuana use among young adolescents. *Journal of Behavioral Medicine*, 10: 559–79.

Harrison, J.A., Mullen, P.D. and Green, L.W. (1992) A meta-analysis of studies of the health belief model with adults. *Health Education Research, Theory and Practice*, 7: 107–16.

Harvey, M.R., Whitmer, R.W., Hilyer, J.C. and Brown, K.C. (1993) The impact of a comprehensive medical benefit cost management program for the City of Birmingham: results at five years. *American Journal of Health Promotion*, 7: 296–303.

Havelock, R. (1974) *Educational Innovation in the United States*, volume 1. Ann Arbor, MI, University of Michigan Report.

Hawe, P. (1994) Capturing the meaning of 'community' in community intervention evaluation: some contributions from community psychology. *Health Promotion International*, 9: 199–210.

Hawkins, M., Gray, C. and Hawkins, C. (1995) Gender differences of reported safer sex behaviours within a random sample of college students. *Psychological Reports*, 77: 963–8.

Haynes, B.R., Sackett, D.L., Taylor, W.D., Gibson, E.S. and Johnson, A.C. (1978) Increased absenteeism from work after detecting and labelling of hypertensive patients. *New England Journal of Medicine*, 148: 1910–13.

Heather, N., Campion, P., Neville, R. and MacCabe, D. (1987) Evaluation of a controlled drinking minimal intervention for problem drinkers in general practice (the DRAMS Scheme). *Journal of the Royal College of General Practitioners*, 37: 358–63.

Hebert, J.R., Harris, D.R., Sorensen, G., Stoddard, A.M., Hunt, M.K. and Morris, D.H. (1993) A work-site nutrition intervention: its effects on the consumption of cancer-related nutrients. *American Journal of Public Health*, 83: 391–3.

Heckhausen, H. (1991) *Motivation and Action*. Berlin: Springer.

Hein, H.O., Suadicani, P. and Gyntelberg, F. (1992) Ischaemic heart disease incidence by social class and form of smoking: the Copenhagen male study – 17 years' follow-up. *Journal of Internal Medicine*, 231: 477–83.

Hennekens, C.H., Rosner, B. and Cole, D.S. (1978) Daily alcohol consumption and fatal coronary disease. *American Journal of Epidemiology*, 107: 196–200.

Her Majesty's Stationery Office (HMSO) (1987) *AIDS Monitoring Responses to Public Education Campaigns. February 1986–February 1987*. London: HMSO.

Hersey, J.C., Klibanoff, L.S., Lam, D.J. and Taylor, R.L. (1984) Promoting social support: the impact of California's friends can be good medicine campaign. *Health Education Quarterly*, 11: 293–311.

Herzlich, C. (1973) *Health and Illness*. London: Academic Press.

Higbee, K. (1969) Fifteen years of fear arousal. Research on threat appeals: 1953–1968. *Psychological Bulletin*, 72: 426–44.

Hingson, R.W., Scotch, N., Mangione, T., Meyers, A., Glantz, L., Heeren, T., Line, M., Mucartel, M. and Pierce, G. (1983) Impact of legislation raising the legal drinking age in Massachusetts from 18 to 20. *American Journal of Public Health*, 73: 163–70.

Holder, H.D. (1987) *Control Issues in Alcohol Abuse Prevention: Strategies for States and Communities*. Advances in Substances Abuse Suppl 1. Greenwich, CT: JAI.

Holland, J., Ramazanoglu, C., Scott, S., Sharpe, S. and Thomson, R. (1990) Sex, gender and power: young women's sexuality in the shadow of AIDS. *Sociology of Health and Illness*, 12: 336–50.

Holmes, T.H. and Rahe, R.H. (1967) The Social Readjustment Rating Scale. *Journal of Psychosomatic Research*, 11: 213–18.

Hovland, C.I., Lumsdaine, A.A. and Sheffield, F.D. (1949) *Experiments on Mass Communication*. Princeton, NJ: Princeton University Press.

Hunt, S.M. and Martin, C.J. (1988) Health-related behavioural change – a test of a new model. *Psychology and Health*, 2: 209–30.

Hunt, S.M., McEwan, J. and McKenna, S.P. (1986) *Measuring Health Status*. London: Croom Helm.

Hunter, D. (1955) *The Diseases of Occupations*. London: Hodder & Stoughton.

Hypertension Prevention Trial (HPT) Research Group (1990) The Hypertension Prevention Trial: three-year effects of dietary changes on blood pressure. *Archives of Internal Medicine*, 150: 153–62.

Ingham, R. and Bennett, P. (1990) Health psychology in community settings: models and methods. In P. Bennett, J. Weinman and P. Spurgeon (eds) *Current Developments in Health Psychology*. London: Harwood Press.

Ingham, R. and Van Zessen, G. (1997) Towards an alternative model of sexual behaviour: from individual properties to interactional processes. In L. van Camphoudt, M. Cohen, G. Guizzardi and D. Hausser (eds) *Sexual Interactions and HIV Risk: New Conceptual Perspectives in European Research*. London: Taylor and Francis.

Irvine, M.J., Johnston, D.W., Jenner, D.A. and Marie, G.V. (1986) Relaxation and stress management in the treatment of essential hypertension. *Journal of Psychosomatic Research*, 30: 437–50.

Iscoe, I. (1974) Community psychology and the competent community. *American Psychologist*, 29: 607–13.

Isen, A.M. (1987) Positive affect, cognitive processes, and social behaviour. In L. Berkowitz (ed.) *Advances in Experimental Social Psychology*, 20. New York: Academic Press.

Israel, B.A. and Shurman, S.J. (1990) Social support, control and the stress process. In K. Glanz, F. Lewis and B. Rimmer (eds) *Health Behaviour and Health Education*. San Francisco: Jossey-Bass.

Ivancevitch, J.M. and Matteson, M.T. (1989) Promoting the individual's health and well-being. In C.L. Copper and R. Payne (eds) *Causes, Coping and Consequences of Stress at Work*. Chichester: Wiley.

Jacobs, D.R. Jr., Luepker, R.V., Mittelmark, M.B. *et al.* (1986) Community-wide prevention strategies: evaluation design of the Minnesota Heart Health Program. *Journal of Chronic Diseases*, 39: 775–88.

Jacobson, B. (1981) *The Lady Killers: Why Smoking Is a Feminist Issue*. London: Pluto Press.

Jacobson, E. (1938) *Progressive Relaxation*. Chicago, IL: University of Chicago.

Janis, I.L. and Feshbach, S. (1953) Effects of fear-arousing communications. *Journal of Abnormal and Social Psychology*, 48: 78–92.

Janis, I.L. and Terwilliger, R. (1962) An experimental study of psychological resistances to fear-arousing communications. *Journal of Abnormal and Social Psychology*, 65: 403–10.

Janz, N. and Becker, M.H. (1984) The health belief model: a decade later. *Health Education Quarterly*, 11: 1–47.

Jarvis, M. (1989) Helping smokers give up. In S. Pearce and J. Wardle (eds) *The Practice of Behavioural Medicine*. Oxford: Oxford Science Publications and the British Psychological Society.

Jason, L.A., Gruder, C.L., Buckenberger, L. *et al.* (1987) A 12-month follow-up of a worksite smoking cessation intervention. *Health Education Research*, 2: 185–94.

Jason, L.A., Gruder, C.L., Martino, S. and Flay, B.R. (1987) Worksite group meetings and the effectiveness of a televised smoking cessation intervention. *American Journal of Community Psychology*, 15: 57–72.

Jeffery R.W. (1995) Community programs for obesity prevention: The Minnesota Heart Health Program. *Obesity Research*, 3: 283–8.

Jeffery, R.W., Forster, J.L. and French, S.A. (1993) The Healthy Worker Project: a work-site intervention for weight control and smoking cessation. *American Journal of Public Health*, 83: 395–401.

Jeffery, R.W., Forster, J.L., Schmid, T., McBride, C., Rooney, B. and Pirie, P. (1990) Community attitudes toward public policies to control alcohol, tobacco and high fat food consumption. *American Journal of Preventive Medicine*, 6: 12–19.

Jeffs, B.W. and Saunders, W.M. (1983) Minimising alcohol related offences by enforcement of the existing licensing legislation. *British Journal of Addiction*, 78: 67–77.

Jenkins, C.D. (1992) Assessment of outcomes of health intervention. *Social Science and Medicine*, 35: 367–75.

Johnson, C.C. and Nicklas, T.A. (1995) Health ahead – The Heart Smart family approach to prevention of cardiovascular disease. *The American Journal of the Medical Sciences*, 310: 127–32.

Johnson, J.V., Stewart, W., Hall, E.M., Fredlund, P. and Theorell, T. (1996) Long-term psychosocial work environment and cardiovascular mortality among Swedish men. *American Journal of Public Health*, 86: 324–31.

Joseph, S.C. (1988) Current issues concerning AIDS in New York City. *New York State Journal of Medicine*, 5: 253–8.

Kahneman, D., Slovic, P. and Tversky, A. (1982) *Judgement Under Uncertainty: Heuristics and Biases*. New York: Cambridge University Press.

Kannel, W.B. (1995) Epidemiologic insights into atherosclerotic cardiovascular disease – from the Framingham Study. In M.L. Pollock and D.H. Schmidt (eds) *Heart Disease and Rehabilitation*. Champaign, IL: Human Kinetics.

Kaplan, B.H. (1975) An epilogue: toward further research on family and health. In B.H. Kaplan and J.C. Cassel (eds) *Family and Health: An Epidemiological Approach*. Chapel Hill, NC: University of North Carolina, Institute for Research and Social Science.

Karasek, R., Baker, D., Marker, F., Ahlbom, A. and Theorell, T. (1981) Job decision latitude, job demands, and cardiovascular disease: a prospective study of Swedish men. *American Journal of Public Health*, 71: 694–705.

Karasek, R. and Theorell, T. (1990) *Healthy work: Stress, Productivity and the Reconstruction of Healthy Life*. New York: Basic Books.

Kasl, S.V. (1980) Cardiovascular risk reduction in a community setting: some comments. *Journal of Consulting and Clinical Psychology*, 48: 143–9.

Kelly, J.A., St Lawrence, J.S., Brasfield, T.L., Lemke, A., Amedei, T., Roffman, R.E., Hood, H.V., Smith, J.E., Kilgore, H. and McNeill, Jr. C. (1990) Psychological factors that predict AIDS high risk versus precautionary behavior. *Journal of Consulting and Clinical Psychology*, 58: 117–20.

Kelly, J.A., Murphy, D.A., Washington, C.D. and Wilson, T.S. (1994) The effects of HIV/AIDS intervention groups for high-risk women in urban clinics. *American Journal of Public Health*, 84: 1918–22.

Kelman, H.C. and Hovland, C.I. (1953) 'Reinstatement' of the communicator in delayed measurement of opinion change. *Journal of Abnormal and Social Psychology*, 48: 326–35.

Kenny, J. (1989) Fear and humour in prevention campaigns. In M. Paalman (ed.) *Promoting safer sex: Prevention of Sexual Transmission of AIDS and Other STDs*. Amsterdam: Swets and Zeitlinger.

Kerr, M. and Charles, N. (1983) *Attitudes to the Feeding and Nutrition of Young Children: Preliminary Report*. York: University of York.

Kessler, R.C. and Neighbors, H.W. (1986) A new perspective on the relationships among race, social class, and psychological distress. *Journal of Health and Social Behavior*, 27: 107–15.

Kieffer, C. (1984) Citizen empowerment: a developmental perspective. *Prevention in Health Services*, 3: 9–36.

Kiloran, A. (1993) Pacemaker. *Health Service Journal*, 103: 26–7.

Klepp, K-I., Halper, A. and Perry, C.L. (1986) The efficacy of peer leaders in drug abuse prevention. *Journal of School Health*, 56: 407–11.

Klepp, K., Ndeki, S., Shea, A. *et al.* (1994) AIDS education for primary school children in Tanzania: an evaluation study. *AIDS*, 8: 1157–62.

Klesges, R.C., Cigrang, J. and Glasgow, R.E. (1989) Worksite smoking modification programs: a state-of-the-art review and directions for future research. In M. Johnston and T. Marteau (eds) *Applications in Health Psychology*. New Brunswick, NJ: Transaction Publishers.

Klesges, R.C., Vasey, B.S. and Glasgow, R.E. (1986) A worksite smoking modification competition: potential for public health impact. *American Journal of Public Health*, 76: 198–200.

Kok, G., Den Boer, D., DeVries, H., Gerrards, F., Hospers, H.J. and Mudde, A.N. (1992) Self efficacy and attribution theory in health education. In R. Schwarzer (ed.) *Self-Efficacy: Thought Control of Action*. Washington DC: Hemisphere.

Kolata, G. (1987) Erotic films in AIDS cut risky behavior. *New York Times*, 3 November, p. 7.

Krantz, D.S. and Durel, L.A. (1983) Psychobiological substrates of the Type A behavior pattern. *Health Psychology*, 2: 393–411.

Lam, W., Size, P., Sacks, H. and Chalmers, T. (1987) Meta-analysis of randomised controlled trials of nicotine chewing-gum. *Lancet*, ii: 27–30.

Lamb, K.L., Brodie, D.A. and Roberts, K. (1988) Physical fitness and health-related fitness as indicators of a positive health state. *Health Promotion International*, 3: 171–82.

Lando, H.A., McGovern, P.G. and Siple, C. (1989) Public service application of an effective clinic approach to smoking cessation. *Health Education Research, Theory and Practice*, 4: 103–9.

Lando, H.A., Pechacek, T.F., Pirie, P.L., Murray, D.M., Mittelmark, M.B., Lichtenstein, E., Nothwehr, F. and Gray, C. (1995) Changes in adult cigarette smoking in the Minnesota Heart Health Program. *American Journal of Public Health*, 85: 201–9.

Langie, J.K. (1977) Social networks, health beliefs and preventive health behavior. *Journal of Health and Social Behavior*, 18: 244–60.

LaPiere, R. (1934) Attitudes versus actions. *Social Forces*, 13: 230–37.

Lau, H. (1975) Cost of alcoholic beverages as a determinant of alcohol consumption. In N. Gibbins, R. Israel, Y. Kalant, H. Popham, R. Schmidt and W. Smart (eds) *Research Advances in Alcohol and Drug Problems*. New York: Wiley.

Lau, R., Kane, R., Berry, S., Ware, J. and Roy, D. (1980) Channeling health: a review of the evaluation of televised health campaigns. *Health Education Quarterly*, 7: 56–87.

Law, M.R., Wald, N.J. and Thompson, S.G. (1994) By how much and how quickly does reduction in serum cholesterol lower risk of ischaemic heart disease? *British Medical Journal*, 308: 367–72.

Lazarfield, P. and Merton, R.K. (1972) Mass communication, popular taste, and organized social action. In W. Schramm and D. Roberts (eds) *The Process and Effects of Mass Communication*. Urbana, Illinois: University of Illinois Press.

Lazarus, R.S. and Folkman, S. (1984) *Stress, Appraisal and Coping*. New York: Springer.

Le Bas, J. (1989) Comprehensibility of patient education literature. *Journal of Psychiatry*, 23: 542–6.

Leathar, D.S. (1981) Lack of response to health guidance amongst heavy drinkers. In M.R. Turner (ed.) *Preventive Nutrition and Society*. London: Academic Press.

Lee, A.M. and Owen, N. (1985) Reasons for discontinuing regular physical activity subsequent to a fitness course. *The ACHPER National Journal*, March: 7–9.

Lefebvre, R. and Flora, J. (1988) Social marketing and public health. *Health Education Quarterly*, 15: 299–315.

Leon, A.S. (1995) Scientific rationale for preventive practices in atherosclerotic and hypertensive cardiovascular disease. In M.L. Pollock and D.H. Schmidt (eds) *Heart Disease and Rehabilitation*. Champaign, IL: Human Kinetics.

Lerman, C., Trock, B., Rimer, B., Boyce, A., Jepson, C. and Engstrom, P. (1991) Psychological and behavioral implications of abnormal mammograms. *Annals of Internal Medicine*, 114: 657–61.

Leventhal, H. and Cleary, P. (1980) The smoking problem: a review of the research and theory in behavioral risk reduction. *Psychological Bulletin*, 88: 370–405.

Leventhal, H., Prochaska, T.R. and Hirshman, R.S. (1985) Preventive health behavior across the lifespan. In J.C. Rosen and L.J. Solomon (eds) *Prevention in Health Psychology*. Hanover, NH: University Press of New England.

Leventhal, H., Safer, M.A., Cleary, P.D. and Gutmann, M. (1980) Cardiovascular risk modification by community-based programs for life-style change: comments on the Stanford study. *Journal of Consulting and Clinical Psychology*, 48: 150–8.

Leventhal, H., Safer, M. and Paganis, D. (1983) The impact of communications on health beliefs, decisions and behaviours. *Health Education Quarterly*, 10: 1–29.

Levi, L. (1974) Psychosocial stress and disease: a conceptual model. In E.K. Gunderson and R.H. Rahe (eds) *Life Stress and Illness*. Springfield, IL: Charles C. Thomas.

Levy, S., Lee, J., Bagley, C. and Lippman, M. (1988) Survival hazards analysis in first recurrent breast cancer patients: seven-year follow-up. *Psychosomatic Medicine*, 50: 520–8.

Levy, S. and Schain, W. (1987) Psychological response and breast cancer: direct and indirect contributions to treatment outcome. In M. Lippman, A. Lichter, and D. Danforth (eds) *Diagnosis and Treatment of Breast Cancer*. New York: Saunders.

Lewis, B., Mann J.I. and Mansini, M. (1986) Reducing the risks of coronary heart disease in individuals and the population. *Lancet*, i: 956–9.

Lewis, K.S. (1994) 'An examination of the health belief model when applied to diabetes mellitus.' Unpublished doctoral dissertation. Sheffield: University of Sheffield.

Lewit, E., Coates, D. and Grossman, M. (1981) The effects of governmental regulation on teenage smoking. *Journal of Law and Economics*, 24: 545–69.

Ley, P. (1988) *Communicating with Patients*. London: Croom Helm.

Ley, P., Jain, V.K. and Skilbeck, C.E. (1976) A method for decreasing patients' medication errors. *Psychological Medicine*, 6: 599–601.

Ley, P. and Llewelyn, S. (1995) Improving patients' understanding, recall, satisfaction and compliance. In A. Broome and S. Llewelyn (eds) *Health Psychology: Processes and Applications*. London: Chapman & Hall.

Li, V.C., Kim, Y.J., Ewart, C.K., Terry, P.B., Cuthie, J.C., Wood, J., Emmett, E.A. and Permutt, S. (1984) Effects of physician counseling on the smoking behavior of asbestos-exposed workers. *Preventive Medicine*, 13: 462–76.

Lichtenstein, E. and Glasgow, R.E. (1992) Smoking cessation: what have we learned over the past decade? *Journal of Consulting and Clinical Psychology*, 60: 518–27.

Liebert, R.M. and Schwertzenberg, N.S. (1977) Effects of mass media. *Annual Review of Psychology*, 28: 141–73.

Linder, D. and Worchel, S. (1970) Opinion change as a result of effortfully drawing a counter-attitudinal conclusion. *Journal of Experimental Social Psychology*, 6: 432–48.

Linegar, J., Chesson, C. and Nice, D. (1991) Physical fitness gains following simple environmental change. *American Journal of Preventive Medicine*, 7: 298–310.

Littlewood, R. and Lipsedge, M. (1988) Psychiatric illness among British Afro-Caribbeans. *British Medical Journal*, 296: 950–1.

Louira, D. (1988) Some concerns about educational approaches in AIDS prevention. In R. Schinazi and A. Nahmias (eds) *AIDS Children, Adolescents and Heterosexual Adults*. New York: Elsevier Science Publications.

Lundberg, U., de Chateau, P., Winberg, J. and Frankenhauser, M. (1981) Catecholamine and cortisol excretion patterns in three year old children and their parents. *Journal of Human Stress*, 7: 3–11.

Maccoby, N. (1988) The community as a focus for health promotion. In S. Spacapan and S. Oskamp (eds) *The Social Psychology of Health*. Newbury Park, CA: Sage.

Macdonald, G. (1992) Communication theory and health promotion. In R. Bunton and G. Macdonald (eds) *Health Promotion Disciplines and Diversity*. London: Routledge.

McDonald, P. and Estep, R. (1985) Prime time drug depictions. *Contemporary Drug Problems*, 14: 419–38.

McGill, H.C. and Stern, M.P. (1979) Sex and atherosclerosis. *Atherosclerosis Review*, 4: 157–248.

McGuire, W. (1985) Attitudes and attitude change. In G. Lindzey and E. Aronson (eds) *Handbook of Social Psychology*, Volume 2. New York: Random House.

McGuire, W.J. (1964) Inducing resistance to persuasion. In L. Berkowitz (ed.) *Advances in Experimental Social Psychology*, Volume 1. New York: Academic Press.

McIlvain, H.E., Thompson, A.V., McKinney, M.E. and Todd, G.L. (1992) Application of the MRFIT smoking cessation program to a healthy, mixed-sex sample. *American Journal of Preventive Medicine*, 8: 165–70.

McKeigue, P.M., Marmot, M.G., Adelstein, A.M., Hunt, S.P., Shipley, M.J., Butler, S.M., Riemersma, R.A. and Turner, P.R. (1985) Diet and risk factors for coronary heart disease in Asians in north-west London. *Lancet*, ii: 1086–90.

Mackie, D., Worth, L. and Asuncion, A. (1990) Processing of persuasive in-group messages. *Journal of Personality and Social Psychology*, 58: 812–22.

McKusick, L., Conant, M.A. and Coates, T.J. (1985) The AIDS epidemic: a model for developing intervention strategies for reducing high risk behaviour in gay men. *Sexually Transmitted Diseases*, 12: 229–34.

McKusick, L., Coates, T.J., Morin, S.F., Pollack, L. and Hoff, N. (1990) Longitudinal predictors of reductions in unprotected anal intercourse among gay men in San Francisco – the AIDS Behavioral Research Project. *American Journal of Public Health*, 80: 978–83.

McMaster, V., Nicholas, S. and Machin, D. (1985) Evaluation of breast self-examination teaching materials in a primary care setting. *Journal of the Royal College of General Practitioners*, 17: 21–3.

McQueen, D. (1987) *Research in Health Behaviour, Health Promotion and Public Health*, working paper. Edinburgh: Research Unit in Health and Behavioural Change.

Maddux, J. and Rogers, R. (1983) Protection motivation and self efficacy. A revised theory of fear appeals and attitude change. *Journal of Experimental Social Psychology*, 19: 464–79.

Maes, S., Kittel, F., Scholten, H. and Verhoeven, C. (in submission) Effects of the Brabantia-project, a Dutch wellness-health programme at the worksite.

Maheswaran, D. and Meyers-Levey, J. (1990) The influence of message framing and issue involvement. *Journal of Marketing Resources*, 27: 361–7.

Maibach, E. (1993) Social marketing for the environment: using information campaigns to promote environmental awareness and behavior change. *Health Promotion International*, 8: 209–24.

Malfetti, J.L. (1985) Public information and education sections of the report of the Presidential Commission on Drunk Driving: A critique and a discussion of research implications. *Accident Analysis and Prevention*, 17: 347–53.

Malow, R.M., West, J.A. and Corrigan, S.A. *et al.* (1994) Outcome of psycho-education for HIV risk reduction. *AIDS Education and Prevention*, 6: 113–25.

Mann, J., Tarantola, D. and Netter, T. (1992) *AIDS in the World.* Cambridge, MA: Harvard University Press.

Mantell, J.E., Kochems, L.M. and Divittis, T. (1987) 'Prevention of immuno-deficiency virus (HIV): AIDS risk reduction interventions with high risk groups.' Paper presented at the annual meeting of the American Public Health Association, New Orleans, LA, March.

Markides, K. (1983) Mortality among minority populations: a review of recent patterns and trends. *Public Health Reports*, 98: 252–60.

Markovtiz, J.H. and Matthews, K.A. (1991) Platelets and coronary heart disease: potential psychophysiologic mechanisms. *Psychosomatic Medicine*, 53: 643–68.

Marlatt, G.A. and Gordon, J.R. (1980) Determinants of relapse: Implications for the maintenance of behavioural change. In P.O. Davidson and S.M. Davidson (eds) *Behavioral Medicine: Changing Health Lifestyles.* New York: Brunner/Mazel.

Marlett, G.A., Baer, J.S. and Quigley, L.A. (1994) Self-efficacy and addictive behaviour. In A. Bandura (ed.) *Self-Efficacy in Changing Societies.* Marbach: Johann Jacobs Foundation.

Marmot, M.G. (1994) Lowering population cholesterol concentrations probably isn't harmful. *British Medical Journal*, 308: 351–2.

Marmot, M.G., Shipley, M.J. and Rose, G. (1984) Inequalities in health – specific explanations of a general pattern? *Lancet*, i: 1003–6.

Marmot, M.G., Davey Smith, G., Stansfield, D., Patel, C., North, F., Head, J., White, I., Brunner, E. and Feeney, A. (1991) Health inequalities among British civil servants: the Whitehall II study. *Lancet*, 337: 1387–92.

Marsh, A. and Matheson, J. (1983) *Smoking Attitudes and Behaviour.* London: HMSO.

Marteau, T.M. (1994) Psychology and screening: narrowing the gap. *British Journal of Clinical Psychology*, 33: 1–10.

Martin, C.J., Platt, S.D. and Hunt, S. (1987) Housing conditions and health. *British Medical Journal*, 294: 1125–7.

Maslow, A.H. (1970) *Motivation and Personality.* New York: Harper and Row.

Matthews, K.A. and Haynes, S.G. (1986) Type A behavior pattern and coronary disease risk: update and critical evaluation. *American Journal of Epidemiology*, 123: 923–60.

Matthews, K.A. and Stoney, C.M. (1988) Influences of sex and age on cardiovascular reponses during stress. *Psychosomatic Medicine*, 50: 46–56.

Mayer, J.A., Jermanovitch, A., Wright, B., Elder, J.P., Drew, J.A. and Williams, S.J. (1994) Changes in health behaviours of older adults: The San Diego Medicare preventive health project. *Preventive Medicine*, 23: 127–33.

Maynard, A. (1985) The role of economic measures in preventing drinking problems. In N. Heather, I. Roberston and P. Davies (eds) *The Misuse of Alcohol: Crucial Issues in Dependence, Treatment and Prevention.* London: Croom Helm.

Mayou, R., Williamson, B. and Foster, A. (1976) Attitudes and advice after myocardial infarction. *British Medical Journal*, 1: 1577–9.

Mead, H. (1934) *Mind, Self and Society*. Chicago, IL: University of Chicago Press.

Meichenbaum, D. (1974) *Cognitive Behaviour Modification*. Morriston, NJ: General Learning Press.

Meichenbaum, D. (1985) *Stress Inoculation Training*. New York: Pergamon.

Mercer, G.W. (1985) The relationships among driving while impaired charges, police drinking-driving roadcheck activity, media coverage and alcohol related casualty traffic accidents. *Accident Analysis Review*, 17: 467–74.

Metson, D., Kassianos, G.C., Norman, D.P. and Moriarty, J.M. (1991) Effect of information leaflets on long-term recall – useful or useless? *The British Journal of Family Planning*, 13: 337–46.

Meyer, A.J., Nash, J.D., McAlister, A.L., Maccoby, N. and Farquhar, J.W. (1980) Skills training in a cardiovascular health education campaign. *Journal of Consulting and Clinical Psychology*, 48: 129–42.

Meyerowitz, B.E. and Chaiken, S. (1987) The effect of message framing on breast self-examination attitudes, intentions and behaviour. *Journal of Personality and Social Psychology*, 52: 500–10.

Milio, N. (1986) *Promoting Health Through Public Policy*. Ottawa: Canadian Public Health Association.

Miller, W.R. (1983) Motivational interviewing with problem drinkers. *Behavioural Psychotherapy*, 11: 147–72.

Miller, W.R. and Rollnick, S. (1991) *Motivational Interviewing: Preparing People to Change Addictive Behavior*. New York: Guilford.

Milne, D. (1992) *Assessment. A Mental Health Portfolio*. Windsor: NFER-Nelson.

Minneker-Hugel, E., Unland, H. and Buchkremer, G. (1992) Behavioural relapse prevention strategies in smoking cessation. *The International Journal of the Addictions*, 27: 627–34.

Mintel (1991) *Children: The Influencing Factor*. London: Mintel International Group Ltd.

Mirowsky, J. and Ross, C.E. (1986) Social patterns of distress. *Annual Review of Sociology*, 12: 23–45.

Moore, L. (1996) *Smoke-Free Pubs. Briefing Review No. 3*. Bristol: Health Promotion Research Programme, University of Bristol.

Mudde, A.A., De Vries, H. and Dolders, M. (1995) Evaluation of a Dutch community-based smoking cessation intervention. *Preventive Medicine*, 24: 61–70.

Muldoon, M.F., Manuck, S.B. and Matthews, K.A. (1991) Mortality experiences in cholesterol reduction trials (correspondence). *New England Journal of Medicine*, 324: 922–3.

Murphy, S. and Bennett, P. (1994) Psychological perspectives on young adults' health behaviour: some implications for health promotion. In G. Penny, P. Bennett and M. Herbert (eds) *Health Psychology: A Lifespan Perspective*. Reading: Harwood Academic Publishers.

Murphy, S. and Smith, C. (1993) Crutches, confetti or useful tools? Professionals, views on and use of health education leaflets. *Health Education Research, Theory and Practice*, 19: 369–83.

Myers, J.K., Lindenthal, J.J. and Pepper, M.P. (1974) Social class, life events, and psychiatric symptoms: a longitudinal study. In B.S. Dohrenwend and B.P. Dohrenwend (eds) *Stressful Life Events: Their Nature and Effects*. New York: Wiley.

Narang, I. and Murphy, S. (1994) An assessment of ante-natal care for Asian women. *British Journal of Midwifery*, 2: 169–74.

National Center for Health Statistics (NCHS) (1988) *AIDS Knowledge and Attitudes for May and June 1988. Advance Data No. 160.* Washington DC: National Academic Press.

National Highway Traffic Safety Administration (1988) *Alcohol Involvement in Fatal Accidents, 1986.* Report No. DOT HS807268. Washington DC: NHSTSA.

National Research Council (NRC) Committee on Diet and Health, Food and Nutrition Board, Commission on Life Sciences (1986) *Diet and Health Implications for Reducing Chronic Disease Risk.* Washington DC: National Academic Press.

Neil, H.A.W., Roe, L., Moore, J.W., Clark, G.M.G., Brown, J., Thorogood, M., Stratton, I.M., Lancaster, T., Mann, D. and Fowler, G.H. (1995) Randomised trial of lipid lowering dietary advice in general practice: the effects on serum lipids, lipoproteins, and antioxidants. *British Medical Journal*, 310: 569–73.

Nettleton, S. and Bunton, R. (1995) Sociological critiques of health promotion. In R. Bunton, S. Nettleton and R. Burrows (eds) *The Sociology of Health Promotion.* London: Routledge.

Newhagen, J. and Reeves, B. (1987) Emotion and memory responses for negative political advertising: a study of television commercials used in the 1988 presidential campaign. In F. Biocca (ed.) *Television and Political Advertising*, volume 1. Hillsdale, NJ: Lawrence Erlbaum.

Norman, P. and Bennett, P. (1996) Health Locus of Control Models. In M. Conner and P. Norman (eds) *Predicting Health Behaviour: Research and Practice with Social Cognition Models.* Milton Keynes: Open University Press.

Norman, P., Bennett, P., Smith, C. and Murphy, S. (in press) Health locus of control, health value, and health behaviour. *Journal of Health Psychology.*

Norman, P. and Conner, M. (1993) The role of social cognition models in predicting attendance at health checks. *Psychology and Health*, 8: 447–62.

Norman, P. and Conner, M. (1996) The role of social cognition models in predicting health behaviours: future directions. In M. Conner and P. Norman (eds) *Predicting Health Behaviour: Research and Practice with Social Cognition Models.* Buckingham: Open University Press.

Norman, P. and Smith, L. (1995) The theory of planned behaviour and exercise: an investigation into the role of prior behaviour, behavioural intentions and attitude variability. *European Journal of Social Psychology*, 25: 403–15.

Nutbeam, D., Smith, C. and Catford, J. (1990) Evaluation on health education: a review of progress, possibilities and problems. *Journal of Epidemiology and Community Health*, 44(2): 83–9.

Nutbeam, D., Smith, C., Murphy, S. and Catford, J. (1993) Maintaining evaluation designs in a long term community based health promotion programme: Heartbeat Wales case study. *Journal of Epidemiology and Community Health*, 47: 127–33.

Oakley, A. (1974) *The Sociology of Housework.* London: Martin Robertson.

Obrist, P. (1981) *Cardiovascular Psychophysiology. A Perspective.* New York: Plenum.

Ockene, J., Kristeller, J., Goldberg, R., Amick, T., Pekow, P., Hosmer, D., Quirk, M. and Kalan, K. (1991) Increasing the efficacy of physician-delivered smoking interventions. A randomized clinical trial. *Journal of General Internal Medicine*, 6: 1–18.

O'Donnell, L.N., Doval, A.S., Duran, R. and O'Donnell, C. (1995) Video-based sexually transmitted disease patient education: its impact on condom acquisition. *American Journal of Public Health*, 85: 817–22.

Ogborne, A.C. and Smart, R.G. (1980) Will restrictions on alcohol advertising reduce consumption? *British Journal of Addiction*, 75: 293–6.

O'Keefe, M.T. (1971) The anti-smoking commercials: a study of television's impact on behaviour. *Public Opinion Quarterly*, 35: 242–8.

O'Leary, A., Goodhart, F., Jemmott, L.S. and Boccher-Lattimore, D. (1992) Predictors of safer sex on the college campus: a social cognitive theory analysis. *Journal of American College Health*, 40: 254–63.

OPCS (1988) Cigarette smoking 1972–1986. *OPCS Monitor 1988. SS 88/1*. London: HMSO.

Oppenheimer, V. (1974) The life-cycle squeeze. *Demography*, 11: 227–45.

Orbell, S., Crombie, I. and Johnston, G. (1995) Social cognition and social structure in the prediction of cervical screening uptake. *British Journal of Health Psychology*, 1: 35–50.

Ornish, D., Brown, S.E., Scherwitz, L.W., Bilings, J.H., Armstrong, W.T., Ports, T.A., McLanahan, S.M., Kirkeeide, R.L., Brand, R.J. and Gould, K.L. (1990) Can life-style changes reverse coronary heart disease? The lifestyle heart trial. *Lancet*, 336: 470–6.

Ostrow, D.G. (1984) Homosexuality and sexually transmitted diseases. In K.K. Holmes and P. Weisner (eds) *Sexually Transmitted Diseases*. New York: McGraw-Hill.

Owen, N., Ewins, A.L. and Lee, C. (1989) Smoking cessation by mail: a comparison of standard and personalized correspondence course formats. *Addictive Behaviors*, 14: 355–63.

OXCHECK Study Group (1994) Effectiveness of health checks conducted by nurses in primary care: results of the OXCHECK study after one year. *British Medical Journal*, 308: 308–12.

Paffenbarger, R.S., Hyde, R.T., Wing, A.L. and Hsiech, C.C. (1986) Physical activity, all cause mortality and longevity of college alumni. *New England Journal of Medicine*, 314: 605–13.

Parcel, G.S., Taylor, W.C., Brink, S.G., Gottlieb, N., Engquist, K., O'Hara, N.M. and Eriksen, M.P. (1989) Translating theory into practice: intervention strategies for the diffusion of a health promotion innovation. *Family and Community Health*, 12: 1–13.

Pavlov, I.P. (1927) *Conditioned reflexes*. Oxford: Oxford University Press.

Payne, Y., Bennett, P. and Harper, P. (1992) 'The psychological impact of carrier screening for cystic fibrosis.' Paper presented at the 3rd European meeting on Psychosocial Aspects of Genetics, Nottingham, July.

Pekurinen, M. (1989) The demand for tobacco products in Finland. *British Journal of Addiction*, 84: 1183–92.

Pelletier, K.R. (1993) A review and analysis of the health and cost-effective outcome studies of comprehensive health promotion and disease prevention programs at the worksite: 1991–1993 update. *American Journal of Health Promotion*, 8: 50–62.

Pentz, M., Brannon, B., Carlin, V., Barrett, E., Mackinnon, D. and Flay, B. (1989) The power of policy: the relationship of smoking policy to adolescent smoking. *American Journal of Public Health*, 79: 857–62.

Perloff, R. (1993) *The Dynamics of Persuasion*. Hove: Laurence Erlbaum Associates.

Perry, C.L., Klepp, K.I. and Halper, A. *et al.* (1986) A process evaluation study of peer leaders in health education. *Journal of School Health*, 56: 62–7.

Peterson, D., Zeger, S., Remington, R. and Anderson, H. (1992) The effect of state cigarette tax increases on cigarette sales 1955 to 1988. *American Journal of Public Health*, 82: 94–6.

Petty, R. and Cacioppo, J. (1986) The elaboration likelihood model of persuasion. In L. Berkowitz (ed.) *Advances in Experimental Social Psychology, volume 19*. Orlando, FL: Academic Press.

Pill, R. and Stott, N. (1985) Preventive procedures and practices among British working class women. *Health Education Research, Theory and Practice*. 1: 111–19.

Pittman, K., Wilson, P., Taylor, A. and Randolph, S. (1992) Making sexuality education and prevention programs relevant for African-American youth. *Journal of School Health*, 62: 339–44.

Pivnick, A. (1993) HIV infection and the meaning of condoms. *Culture, Medicine and Psychiatry*, 17: 431–53.

Plotnikoff, R.C. and Higginbotham, N. (1995) Predicting low-fat diet intentions and behaviors for the prevention of coronary heart disease: an application of protection motivation theory among an Australian population. *Psychology and Health*, 10: 397–408.

Price, V.A. (1988) Research and clinical issues in treating Type A behavior. In B.K. Houston and C.R. Synder (eds) *Type A Behavior Pattern: Research, Theory, and Practice*. Wiley: New York.

Primm, B. (1987) AIDS: a special report. In J. Dewart (ed.) *The State of Black America 1987*. New York: National Urban League.

Prochaska, J.O. and DiClemente, C.C. (1984) *The Transtheoretical Approach: Crossing Traditional Boundaries of Change*. Homewood, IL: Irwin.

Prochaska, R., DiClemente, C. and Velicer, W. (1988) Comparative analysis of self-help programs for four stages of smoking cessation. Four National Cancer Institute funded self-help smoking cessation trials. Symposium at the Annual Association for the Advancement of Behavior Therapy Convention, New York.

Puska, P., Nissinen, A., Tuomilehto, J., Salonen, J.T., Koskela, K., McAlister, A., Kottke, T.E., Maccoby, N. and Farquhar, J.W. (1985) The community-based strategy to prevent coronary heart disease: conclusions from the ten years of the North Karelia Project. *Annual Review of Public Health*, 6: 147–93.

Quirk, M., Godkin, M. and Schwenzfeier, E. (1993) Evaluation of two AIDS prevention interventions for inner-city adolescent and young adult women. *American Journal of Preventive Medicine*, 9: 21–6.

Ramirez, A. and Lasater, T. (1977) Ethnicity of communicator, self esteem and reactions to fear communications. *Journal of Social Psychology*, 102: 79–91.

Randall, D.M. and Wolff, J.A. (1994) The time interval in the intention-behaviour relationship: meta-analysis. *British Journal of Social Psychology*, 33: 405–18.

Rappaport, J. (1981) In praise of paradox: a social policy of empowerment over prevention. *American Journal of Community Psychology*, 9: 1–25.

Ratneshwar, S. and Chaiken, S. (1991) Comprehension's role in persuasion: the case of its moderating effect on the persuasive impact of source cues. *Journal of Consumer Research*, 18: 52–62.

Reddy, D.M., Fleming, R. and Adesso, V.J. (1992) Gender and health. In S. Maes, H. Leventhal and M. Johnston (eds) *International Review of Health Psychology, Volume 1*. Chichester: Wiley.

Redman, S., Sanson Fisher, R., Kreft, S., Fleming, J. and Dickinson, J. (1995) Is the Australian National Heart Foundation programme effective in reducing cholesterol levels among general practice patients? *Health Promotion International*, 10: 293–303.

Review Panel (1981) Coronary-prone behavior and heart disease: a critical review. *Circulation*, 63: 1199–215.

Rhodes, F. and Wolitski, B. (1990) Perceived effectiveness of fear appeals in AIDS education: relationship to ethnicity, gender, age and group membership. *AIDS Education and Prevention*, 2: 1–11.

Richards, J., Fisher, P. and Conner, F. (1989) The warnings on cigarette packages are ineffective. *Journal of the American Medical Association*, 261: 45.

Richmond, R., Harris, K. and de Almeida Neto, A. (1994) The transdermal nicotine patch: results of a randomised placebo-controlled trial. *The Medical Journal of Australia*, 161: 130–5.

Richmond, R., Heather, N., Wodak, A., Kehoe, L. and Webster, I. (1995) Controlled evaluation of a general practice-based brief intervention for excessive drinking. *Addiction*, 90: 119–32.

Richwald, G.A., Wamsley, M.A., Coulson, A.H. and Moriskey, D.E. (1988) Are condom instructions readable? Results of a readability study. *Public Health Reports*, 103: 355–9.

Rigby, K., Brown, M., Anganostou, P., Ross, M.W. and Rosser, B.R.S. (1989) Shock tactics to counter AIDS: the Australian experience. *Psychology and Health*, 3: 145–59.

Riley, D. (1987) Drink-driving and the alcohol beverage industry: will reducing per capita consumption solve the problem in the United Kingdom? *Accident Analysis and Prevention*, 19: 449–62.

Rippetoe, P.A. and Rogers, R.W. (1987) Effects on components of protection motivation theory on adaptive and maladaptive copings with a health threat. *Journal of Personality and Social Psychology*, 52: 596–604.

Robert, B. and Rosser, S. (1990) Evaluation of the efficacy of AIDS education interventions for homosexually active men. *Health Education Research, Theory and Practice*, 5: 299–308.

Robertson, L.S. (1976) 'Whose behaviour in what marketplace?' Paper presented at the Steinhart Conference on Consumer Behaviour in the Health Marketplace. University of Nebraska, Lincoln, NB, March.

Robinson, J. (1984) Racial inequality and the probability of occupation-related injury or illness. *Milbank Memorial Fund Quarterly*, 62: 567–90.

Robinson, J. and McArthur, L. (1982) Impact of salient vocal qualities on casual attribution for a speaker's behaviour. *Journal of Personality and Social Psychology*, 43: 236–47.

Rogers, C.R. (1951) *Client Centered Therapy*. Boston, MA: Houghton Mifflin.

Rogers, C.R. (1967) *The Therapeutic Relationship and Its Impact*. Madison, WI: University of Wisconsin Press.

Rogers, E. (1983) Diffusion of innovations. New York: Free Press, Macmillan.

Roland, M. and Dixon, M. (1989) Randomised controlled trial of an educational booklet for patients presenting with back pain in general practice. *Journal of the Royal College of General Practitioners*, 39: 244–6.

Rollnick, S., Heather, N. and Bell, A. (1992) Negotiating behaviour change in medical settings: the development of brief motivational interviewing. *Journal of Mental Health*, 1: 25–37.

Ronis, D.L. and Harel, Y. (1989) Health beliefs and breast examination behaviour: analysis of linear structural relations. *Psychology and Health*, 3: 259–85.

Rose, G., Heller, R.F., Pedoe, H.T. and Christie, D.G.S. (1980) Heart Disease Prevention Project: a randomised controlled trial in industry. *British Medical Journal*, 280: 747–51.

Rosen, T.M., Terry, N. and Leventhal, H. (1982) The role of self esteem and coping in response to a threat communication. *Journal of Research in Personality*, 16: 90–107.

Rosenbaum, P. and O'Shea, R. (1992) Large-scale study of Freedom From Smoking clinics – factors in quitting. *Public Health Reports*, 107: 150–5.

Rosenberg, M. (1965) *Society and the Adolescent Self-Image*. Princeton, NJ: Princeton University Press.

Rosenman, R.H. (1978) The interview method of assessment of the coronary-prone behavior pattern. In T.M. Dembroski, S.M. Weiss, J.L. Shields, S.G. Haynes and M. Feinleib (eds) *Coronary-prone behavior*. New York: Springer.

Rosenman, R.H., Brand, R.J., Friedman, M., Straus, R. and Wurm, M. (1975) Coronary heart disease in the Western Collaborative Group Study: final follow-up experience of 8½ years. *Journal of the American Medical Association*, 233: 872–7.

Ross, L.H., Kleffe, H. and McCleary, R. (1987) Liberalisation and drunk-driving laws in Scandinavia. *Accident Analysis and Prevention*, 16: 471–87.

Ross, M.G. and Lappin, B.W. (1967) Community organization: theory, principles and practice. New York: Harper Row.

Rotter, J.B. (1966) Generalised expectancies for internal and external control of reinforcement. *Psychological Monographs*, 80 (609): 1–28.

Royal College of General Practitioners (1986) *Alcohol – A Balanced View. Report from General Practice*. London: Royal College of Practitioners.

Royal College of Psychiatrists (1986) *Alcohol, Our Favourite Drug*. London: Tavistock.

Rudd, P., Price, M.G., Graham, L.E., Beilstein, B.A., Tarbell, S.J.H., Bachetti, P. and Fortmann, S.P. (1986) Consequences of worksite hypertension screening. *American Journal of Medicine*, 80: 853–60.

Russell, M.A.H., Wilson, C. and Baker, C.D. (1979) Effect of general practitioners' advice against smoking. *British Medical Journal*, 2: 231–5.

Ryan, W. (1976) *Blaming the victim*. New York: Vintage Books.

St Lawrence, J. (1993) African American adolescents' knowledge, health related attitudes, sexual behavior and contraceptive decisions: implications for the prevention of adolescent HIV infection. *Journal of Consulting and Clinical Psychology*, 61: 104–12.

St Lawrence, J.S., Jefferson, K.W., Alleyne, E. and Brasfield, T.L. (1995) Comparison of education versus behavioral skills training interventions in lowering sexual HIV-risk behavior of substance-dependent adolescents. *Journal of Consulting and Clinical Psychology*, 63: 154–7.

Sales, J., Duffy, J., Plant, M. and Peck, D. (1989) Alcohol consumption, cigarette sales and mortality in the United Kingdom: an analysis of the period 1970–1985. *Drug and Alcohol Dependence*, 24: 155–60.

Sallis, J.F. and Hovell, M.F. (1990) Determinants of exercise behaviour. *Exercise and Sports Sciences Reviews*, 1: 307–30.

Salonen, J.T. (1987) Did the North Karelia project reduce coronary mortality? *Lancet*, August, 1, 269.

Sarason, S.B. (1974) *A Psychological Sense of Community. Prospects for a Community Psychology.* San Francisco, CA: Jossey-Bass.

Sawyer, R. and Beck, K. (1991) Effects of videotapes on perceived susceptibility to HIV/AIDS among university freshmen. *Health Values*, 15: 31–40.

Schaefer, W. (1987) *Stress Management for Wellness.* New York: Holt, Rhinehart & Winston.

Schaps, E., DiBartolo, R., Moskowitz, J., Palley, C.S. and Churgin, S. (1981) A review of 127 drug abuse prevention program evaluations. *Journal of Drug Issues*, Winter: 17–43.

Schnelle, J.F., Weather, M.G., Hannah, J.T. and Nees, M.C. (1975) Community social evaluation: a multiple baseline analysis of the effects of a legalized liquor law in four middle Tennessee counties. *Journal of Community Psychology*, 3: 224–31.

Schofield, M. and Edwards, K. (1995) Community attitudes to bans on smoking in licensed premises. *Australian Journal of Public Health*, 19: 399–402.

Schwarzer, R. (1992) Self-efficacy in the adoption and maintenance of health behaviors: theoretical approaches and a new model. In R. Schwarzer (ed.) *Self-Efficacy: Thought Control of Action.* Washington DC: Hemisphere.

Schwarzer, R. (1994) Optimism, vulnerability, and self-beliefs as health-related cognitions: a systematic overview. *Psychology and Health*, 9: 161–80.

Scollay, P., Doucett, M., Perry, M. and Winterbottom, B. (1992) AIDS education of college students: the effect of an HIV-positive lecturer. *AIDS Education and Prevention*, 4: 160–71.

Scott, E. and Anderson, P. (1991) Randomized controlled trial of general practitioner intervention in women with excessive alcohol consumption. *Drug and Alcohol Review*, 10: 313–21.

Selye, H. (1956) *The stress of life.* New York: McGraw-Hill.

Sheeran, P. and Abraham, C. (1996) The health belief model. In M. Conner and P. Norman (eds) *Predicting Health Behaviour.* Buckingham: Open University Press.

Shekelle, R.B., Gale, M. and Norusis, M. for the Aspirin Myocardial Infarction Study Research Group (1985) Type A score (Jenkins Activity Survey) and risk of recurrent disease in the Aspirin Myocardial Infarction Study. *American Journal of Cardiology*, 56: 221–5.

Sheppard, B.H., Hartwick, J. and Warshaw, P.R. (1988) The theory of reasoned action: a meta-analysis of past research with recommendations for modifications and future research. *Journal of Consumer Research*, 15: 325–39.

Sherif, C. (1961) *Intergroup Conflict and Cooperation: The Robbers' Cave Experiment.* Oklahoma: Oklahoma Book Exchange.

Sherif, M. and Hovland, C. (1961) *Social Judgement: Assimilation and Contrast Effects in Communication and Attitude Change.* New Haven, CT: Yale University Press.

Shiffman, S. (1986) A cluster-analytic classification of smoking relapse episodes. *Addictive Behaviors*, 11: 295–307.

Shipley, R.H., Orleans, C.T., Wilbur, C.S., Piserchia, M.S. and McFadden, D.W. (1988) Effect of the Johnson & Johnson Live for Life Program on employee smoking. *Preventive Medicine*, 17: 25–34.

Simons-Morton, B.G., Parcel, G.S., O'Hara, N.M., Blair, S.N. and Pate, R.R. (1988) Health-related physical fitness in childhood: status and recommendations. In L. Breslow, J.E. Fielding and L.B. Lave (eds) *Annual Review of Public Health* (volume 9). Palo Alto, CA: Annual Reviews.

Skinner, B.F. (1953) *Science and Human Behavior.* New York: Macmillan.

Slater, M.D. and Flora, J.A. (1991) Health lifestyles: audience segmentation analysis for public health interventions. *Health Education Quarterly*, 18: 221–33.

Slenker, S.E., Price, J.H. and O'Connell, J.K. (1985) Health locus of control of joggers and non-exercisers. *Perceptual and Motor Skills*, 61: 323–8.

Sleutjes, M. (1990) Promoting safer sex among ethnic minority groups. Lifting the real barriers. In M. Paalman (ed.) *Promoting Safer Sex: Prevention of Sexual Transmission of AIDS and other STDs*. Amsterdam: Swets and Zeitlinger.

Smart, R. and Fejer, D. (1974) The effects of high and low fear messages about drugs. *Journal of Drug Education*, 4: 225–35.

Smart, R.G. (1988) Does alcohol advertising affect overall consumption? A review of empirical studies. *Journal of Studies on Alcohol*, 49: 314–23.

Smart, R.G. and Docherty, D. (1976) Effects of the introduction of on-premise drinking on alcohol-related accidents and impaired driving. *Journal of Studies of Alcohol*, 37: 683–6.

Smith, A. and Jacobson, B. (1988) *The Nation's Health. A Strategy for the 1990s*. London: King's Fund.

Smith, C., Roberts, J.L. and Pendelton, L.L. (1988) Booze on the box. The portrayal of alcohol on British television: a content analysis. *Health Education Research*, 3: 267–72.

Smith, C., Nutbeam, D, Roberts, C. and Macdonald, G. (1992) The health promoting school: Progress and future challenges in Welsh secondary schools. *Health Promotion International*, 7: 171–80.

Smith, C., Moore, L. and Trickey, H. (1994) *Community-Based Cardiovascular Disease Prevention: A Review of the Effectiveness of Health Education and Health Promotion*. Utrecht: International Union for Health Promotion and Health Education.

Smith, D.W. (1987) Barriers to risk reduction in a southern community. In D.G. Ostrow (ed.) *Biobehavioral Control of AIDS*. New York: Irvington Publishers.

Soames-Job, R.F. (1988) Effective and ineffective use of fear in health promotion campaigns. *American Journal of Public Health*, 78: 163–7.

Sobo, E.J. (1993) Inner-city women and AIDS: the psycho-social benefits of unsafe sex. *Culture, Medicine and Psychiatry*, 17: 455–85.

Solomon, M.Z. and DeJong, W. (1986) Recent STD prevention efforts and their implications for AIDS health education. *Health Education Quarterly*, 13: 301–16.

Sorensen, G., Morris, D.M., Hunt, M.K., Hebert, J.R., Harris, D.R., Stoddard, A. and Ockene, J.K. (1992) Work-site nutrition intervention and employees' dietary habits: the Treatwell Program. *American Journal of Public Health*, 82: 877–80.

Sorrentino, R.M., Bobocel, D.R., Gitta, M.Z., Olson, J.M. and Hewitt, E.C. (1988) Uncertainty orientation and persuasion: individual differences in the effects of personal relevance on social judgements. *Journal of Personality and Social Psychology*, 55: 357–71.

Stacy, A.W., Sussman, S., Dent, C.W., Burton, D. and Flay, B.R. (1992) Moderators of peer social influence in adolescent smoking. *Personality and Social Psychology Bulletin*, 18: 163–72.

Stacy, R.D. and Lloyd, B.H. (1990) An investigation of beliefs about smoking among diabetes patients: information for improving cessation efforts. *Journal of Patient Education and Counselling*, 15: 181–9.

Stainton Rogers, W. (1991) *Explaining Health and Illness: An Exploration of Diversity*. Hemel Hempstead: Wheatsheaf.

Stamler, R. (1990) The blood pressure problem: risks and their reduction. *Cardiovascular Risk Factors*, 1: 71–9.

Stamler, R., Stamler, J., Grimm, R., Gosch, F.C., Elmer, P. and Dyer, A. (1986) Nutritional therapy for high blood pressure: final report of a four-year randomized trial – the Hypertension Control Program. *Journal of the American Medical Association*, 7: 1484–91.

Stamler, R., Stamler, J., Gosch, F.C., Civinelli, J., Fishman, J. and McKeever, P. (1989) Primary prevention of hypertension by nutritional-hygienic means: final report of a randomized, controlled trial. *Journal of the American Medical Association*, 262: 1801–7.

Steele, P.D. and Thomas, L.A. (1978) Substance abuse and the work place with special attention to employee assistance programs: an overview. *Journal of Applied Behavioural Science*, 24, 4: 315–25.

Steinberg, D. (1979) Metabolism of lipoprotein at the cellular level in relation to atherogenesis. In N.E. Miller and B. Lewis (eds) *Lipoproteins, Atherosclerosis and Coronary Heart Disease*. Amsterdam: Elsevier.

Steptoe, A., Wardle, J., Vinck, J., Tuomisto, M., Holte, A. and Wickstrom, L. (1994) Personality and attitudinal correlates of healthy and unhealthy lifestyles in young adults. *Psychology and Health*, 9: 331–43.

Stiff, J., McCormack, M., Zook, E., Stein, T. and Henry, R. (1990) Learning about AIDS and HIV transmission in college-age students. *Communication Research*, 17: 743–53.

Stoate, H. (1989) Can health screening damage your health? *Journal of the Royal College of General Practitioners*, 39: 193–5.

Stretcher, V., Deveillis, B., Becker, M. and Rosenstock, I. (1986) The role of self efficacy in achieving health behaviour change. *Health Education Quarterly*, 13: 301–16.

Struckman-Johnson, C., Gilliland, R., Struckman-Johnson, D. and North, T. (1990) The effect of fear of AIDS and gender on responses to fear-arousing condom advertisements. *Journal of Applied Social Psychology*, 20: 1396–410.

Stull, D.E. (1987) Conceptualization and measurement of well-being: implications for policy evaluation. In E.F. Borgatta and R.J.V. Montgomery (eds) *Critical Issues in Ageing Policy*. Beverly Hills, CA: Sage Publications.

Sussman, S., Dent, C.W., Simon, T.R., Stacy, A.W., Galaif, E.R., Moss, M.A., Craig, S. and Johnson, C.A. (1995) Immediate impact of social influence-oriented substance abuse prevention curricula in traditional and continuation high schools. *Drugs and Society*, 8: 65–81.

Sutton, S. (1989) Smoking attitudes and behaviour: an application of Fishbein and Ajzen's theory of reasoned action to prediciting and understanding smoking decisions. In T. Ney and A. Gale (eds) *Smoking and Human Behaviour*. Chichester: Wiley.

Tabak, E. (1988) Encouraging patient question asking: a clinical trial. *Patient Education and Counselling*, 12: 37–49.

Tate, J.C., Schmitz, J.M. and Stanton, A.L. (1991) 'Expectancies for smoking withdrawal symptoms: objective assessment of "smoker's lore".' Paper presented at the 12th Annual Scientific Session of the Society of Behavioral Medicine. Washington DC, April.

Taylor, C.B., Farquhar, J.W., Nelson, E. and Agras, S. (1977) Relaxation therapy and high blood pressure. *Archives of General Psychiatry*, 34: 339–42.

Taylor, S.E. (1989) *Positive Illusions: Creative Self-Deception and the Healthy Mind.* New York: Basic Books.

Taylor, V. (1990) Health education: a theoretical mapping. *Health Education Journal,* 49: 13–14.

Terborg, J.R., Hibbard, J. and Glasgow, R.E. (1995) Behavior change at the work-site: does social support make a difference? *American Journal of Health Promotion,* 10: 125–31.

Terry, D.A., Galligan, R.F. and Conway, V.J. (1993) The prediction of safe sex behaviour: the role of intentions, attitudes, norms and control beliefs. *Psychology and Health,* 8: 355–68.

Thoits, P.A. (1982) Conceptual, methodological and theoretical problems in studying social support as a buffer against life stress. *Journal of Health and Social Behavior,* 23: 145–59.

Thomas, M., Goddard, E., Hickman, M. and Hunter, P. (1992) *General Household Survey.* London: HMSO.

Thompson, B., Fries, E., Hopp, H.P., Bowen, D.J. and Croyle, R.T. (1995) The feasibility of a proactive stepped care model for worksite smoking cessation. *Health Education Research, Theory and Practice,* 10: 455–65.

Tonnes, K.M.A. (1990) Why theorise? Ideology in health education. *Health Education Journal,* 49: 2–6.

Tonnes, K. and Tilford, S. (1994) *Health Education: Effectiveness, Efficiency and Equity.* (2nd edn). London: Chapman and Hall.

Townsend, P. and Davidson, N. (eds) (1988) *Inequalities in Health: The Black Report.* London: Penguin Books.

Tudiver, F., Myers, T., Kurtz, R.G., Orr, K., Rowe, C., Jackson, E. and Bullock, S.L. (1992) The talking sex project: Results of a randomized controlled trial of small-group AIDS education for 612 gay and bisexual men. *Evaluation and the Health Professions,* 15(4): 26–42.

Tversky, A. and Kahneman, D. (1982) Judgement under uncertainty: heuristics and biases. In D. Kahneman, P. Slovic and A. Tversky (eds) *Judgement Under Uncertainty: Heuristics and Biases.* New York: Cambridge University Press.

United Nations (1990) *Demographic Yearbook, 1988. Special Topic: Population Census Statistics.* New York: Department of International, Economic and Social Affairs, Statistical Office.

United States Bureau of Census (USBC) (1989) *Statistical Abstract of the United States* (109th edn). Washington DC: US Government Printing Office.

United States Department of Health and Human Services (USDHHS) (1988) *The Surgeon General's Report on Nutrition and Health.* Washington DC: US Government Printing Office.

United States Department of Health and Human Services (USDHHS) (1993) *1992 National Survey of Worksite Health Promotion Activities.* Washington DC: Office of Disease Prevention and Health Promotion.

Valdiserri, R.O., Lyter, D., Leviton, L.C., Callahan, C.M., Kingsley, L.A. and Rinaldo, C.R. (1988) Variables influencing condom use in a cohort of gay and bisexual men. *American Journal of Public Health,* 78: 801–5.

van den Putte, H. (1993) 'On the theory of reasoned action'. Unpublished doctoral thesis, University of Amsterdam.

Van der Velde, F.W., Van der Pligt, J. and Hooykas, C. (1992) Risk perception and behavior: pessimism, realism, and optimism about AIDS-related health behaviour. *Psychology and Health*, 6: 23–38.

Van Iwaarden, M.J. (1985) Public health aspects of the marketing of alcoholic drinks. In M. Grant (ed.) *Alcohol Policies*. Copenhagen: WHO.

Vitaliano, P.P., Russo, J., Carr, J.E., Maiuro, R.D. and Becker, J. (1985) The Ways of Coping Checklist: revision and psychometric qualities. *Multivariate Behavioral Research*, 20: 3–26.

Wadden, T.A. (1984) Relaxation therapy for essential hypertension: specific or non-specific effects. *Journal of Psychosomatic Research*, 28: 53–61.

Wagenaar, A.C. (1983) *Alcohol, Young Drivers and Traffic Accidents*. Lexington, MA: Lexington Books.

Wald, N.J., Nanchahal, K., Thompson, S.G. and Cuckle, H. (1986) Does breathing other people's tobacco smoke cause lung cancer? *British Medical Journal*, 293: 1217–21.

Wallack, L.M. (1980) Mass media campaigns: the odds against finding behavior change. *Health Education Quarterly*, 1: 209–60.

Wallack, L., Breed, W. and Cruz, J. (1987) Alcohol on prime-time television. *Journal for the Study of Alcohol*, 48: 33–8.

Wallston, K.A. and Smith, M.S. (1994) Issues of control and health: the action is in the interaction. In G. Penny, P. Bennett and M. Herbert (eds) *Health Psychology: A Lifespan Perspective*. London: Harwood.

Wallston, K.A. and Wallston, B.S. (1984) Social psychological models of health behavior: an examination and integration. In A. Baum, S. Taylor and J.E. Singer (eds) *Handbook of Psychology and Health, vol. IV: Social aspects of health*. Hillsdale, NJ: Lawrence Erlbaum.

Wallston, K.A., Wallston, B.S. and DeVellis, R. (1978) Development of the multidimensional health locus of control. *Health Education Monographs*, 6: 160–70.

Waterson, E.J., Evans, C. and Murray-Lyon, I.M. (1990) Is pregnancy a time of changing drinking and smoking patterns for fathers as well as mothers? An initial investigation. *British Journal of Addiction*, 85: 389–96.

Waterson, E.J. and Murray-Lyon, I.M. (1989) Alcohol, smoking and pregnancy: some observations on ethnic minorities in the United Kingdom. *British Journal of Addiction*, 84: 323–5.

Watt, G.C.M. and Ecob, R. (1992) Mortality in Glasgow and Edinburgh: a paradigm of inequality in health. *Journal of Epidemiology and Community Health*, 46: 498–505.

Watts, J. (1968) The role of vulnerability in resistance to fear arousing communications. *Dissertation Abstracts International*, 28: 427A.

Weinstein, N.D. (1980) Unrealistic optimism about future life events. *Journal of Personality and Social Psychology*, 39: 806–820.

Weinstein, N. (1984) Why it won't happen to me: perceptions of risk factors and susceptibility. *Health Psychology*, 3: 431–57.

Weiss, G.L. and Larsen, D.L. (1990) Health value, health locus of control and the prediction of health protective behaviors. *Social Behavior and Personality*, 18: 121–36.

Weisse, C., Turbiasz, A. and Whitney, D. (1995) Behavioural training and AIDS risk reduction: overcoming barriers to condom use. *AIDS Education and Prevention*, 7: 50–9.

Wenger, N.S., Kusseling, F.S. and Shapiro, M.F. (1995) Misunderstanding of 'safer sex' by heterosexually active adults. *Public Health Reports*, 110: 618–21.

Werner, E. and Smith, R. (1982) *Vulnerable But Invincible: A Longitudinal Study of Resilient Children and Youth*. New York: McGraw-Hill.

Westman, M., Eden, D. and Shirom, A. (1985) Job stress, cigarette smoking and cessation: conditioning effects of peer support. *Social Science and Medicine*, 20: 637–44.

Whelan, A., Murphy, S. and Smith, C. (1993) *Performance indicators in health promotion: a review of possibilities and problems Technical Report no. 2*. Cardiff: Health Promotion Wales.

Whitehead, M. (1988) *The Health Divide*. Harmondsworth: Penguin.

Whitehead, W.E. (1992) Behavioral medicine approaches to gastrointestinal disorders. *Journal of Consulting and Clinical Psychology*, 60: 605–12.

Wicke, D.M., Lorge, R.E., Coppin, R.J. and Jones, K.P. (1994) The effectiveness of waiting room notice-boards as a vehicle for health education. *Family Practice*, 11: 292–5.

Wilbur, C.S., Zifferblatt, S.M., Pinsky, J.L. and Zifferblatt, J. (1981) Healthy vending: a cooperative pilot research program to stimulate good health in the marketplace. *Preventive Medicine*, 10: 85–93.

Wilder, D.A. (1990) Some determinants of the persuasive power of in-groups and out-groups: organization of information and attribution of independence. *Journal of Personality and Social Psychology*, 59: 1202–13.

Wilkinson, C., Jones, J.M. and McBride, J. (1990) Anxiety caused by abnormal result of cervical smear test: a controlled trial. *British Medical Journal*, 300: 440.

Wilkinson, M. (1992) Income distribution and life expectancy. *British Medical Journal*, 304: 165–8.

Williams, D.R. (1990) Socioeconomic differentials in health: a review and redirection. *Social Psychology Quarterly*, 53(2): 81–99.

Williams, T. and de Panafieu, C. (1985) *School Health Education in Europe*. Southampton: University of Southampton, Health Education Unit.

Winett, R.A. (1995) A framework for health promotion and disease prevention programs. *American Psychologist*, May: 341–51.

Winett, R.A., King, A.C. and Altman, D.G. (1989) *Health Psychology and Public Health. An Integrative Approach*. New York: Pergamon.

Wolcott, D.L., Sullivan, G. and Klein, D. (1990) Longitudinal change in HIV transmission risk behaviours by gay male physicians. *Journal of Psychosomatics*, 31: 159–67.

Woolfolk, R. and Lehrer, P. (eds) (1993) *Principles and Practice of Stress Management*. (2nd edn) New York: Guilford.

World Health Organization (WHO) (1958) *The First Ten Years. The Health Organization*. Geneva: WHO.

World Health Organization (WHO) (1986) *Ottawa Charter for Health Promotion*. Ottawa: WHO.

World Health Organization (WHO) (1988) *Towards Healthy Public Policies on Alcohol and Other Drugs*. Consensus Statement proposed by WHO Expert Working Group, Sydney–Canberra. Geneva: WHO.

World Health Organization (WHO) (1990) *Diet, Nutrition, and the Prevention of Chronic Diseases. WHO Technical Report 797*. Geneva: WHO.

World Health Organization (WHO) (1991) *Supportive Environments for Health. The Sundsvall Statement*. Geneva: WHO.

Wu, C. and Shaffer, D. (1987) Susceptibility to persuasive appeals as a function of source credibility and prior experience with attitude object. *Journal of Personality and Social Psychology*, 52: 677–88.

Yates, F. and Hebblethwaite, D. (1983) A review of the problems prevention approach to drinking problems and an alternative programme which makes use of natural resources within the community. *British Journal of Addiction*, 78: 355–64.

Zelman, D.C., Brandon, T.H., Jorenby, D.E. and Baker, T.B. (1992) Measures of affect and nicotine dependence predict differential response to smoking cessation. *Journal of Consulting and Clinical Psychology*, 60: 943–52.

Zimmerman, M.A. (1990) Taking aim on empowerment research: on the distinction between individual and psychological conceptions. *American Journal of Community Psychology*, 18: 169–74.

Zimmerman, R.S. and Connor, C. (1989) Health promotion in context: the effects of significant others on health behavior change. *Health Education Quarterly*, 16: 57–75.

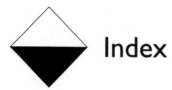 Index

communication theory
  fear appeals, 103–5
  message content, 102–5
  receiver characteristics, 105–6
  source characteristics, 101–2
community interventions, 98, 127
  and cancer, 124–5
  and CHD, 120–4
  and HIV, 125–6
community participation, 144
community psychology, 144
condom use, 28, 42, 43, 83
  and fear arousal, 103–4
  and health belief model, 35
  and HIV transmission, 70
  leaflets, 31
  and locus of control, 31
  and theory of reasoned action/
    planned behaviour, 34
  see also HIV; safer sex
coping, 20, 42, 57, 58, 62, 73, 90, 100
  blunting, 105
  and cigarette smoking, 55, 56, 76,
    78
  and cognitive interventions, 60
  emotion-focused, 19
  monitoring, 105
  problem-focused, 19
coronary heart disease
  aetiology, 17, 20–1
  and community programmes,
    prevention, 120–4
  and screening, 66–9, 73–4
  and self-help, 65–6
  and worksite programmes, 115–18
counselling
  and CHD, 72–5
  and HIV, 70–2
  problem solving approach, 51–4
  and screening, 64, 68
  and smoking cessation, 55–7, 75–8
  stage model, 48
  and stress management, 57–62

diathesis-stress model, 18
DiClemente, 37, 41, 48, 73, 110
diet
  and cancer, 8
  choice, 41, 43

and ethnicity, 15, 133
and health, 8
modification, 22, 67, 74, 75, 95
  in community, 120, 124
  at worksite, 117–19
and protection motivation theory,
  105
recommendations, 7
diffusion of innovations, 83, 106–8,
  111–12, 113, 122
drink-driving, see alcohol
drugs, illicit, 28, 93–4
dual process model, 99

efficacy beliefs, 28–9, 30, 39–40, 43,
  52–3, 71, 83, 144–5
  and communication theory, 104,
    105, 126
  elaboration likelihood model, 100–1,
    102, 103, 105
  and modelling, 120
  and protection motivation theory,
    100
Egan, 52, 53, 54, 57, 63, 69, 74, 146
empowerment, 144–5
environment, 7, 15, 19, 23–4, 43, 47,
  64, 78, 96, 131–4, 136, 144, 145
  and gender, 13
  physical, 14, 134
  social, 134–7
  supportive, 81–2
ethnicity
  and behaviour, 15–16, 134
  and discrimination, 16, 134
  and health, 15–16
  and mortality, 15
  and SES, 16, 134
exchange theory, 109
exercise, 24, 135, 136
  and gender, 24, 135, 136
  and health, 10, 143
  and health locus of control, 31
  manipulating, 67, 68, 74, 86, 95–6,
    115, 119, 123–4, 137
  prevalence, 11
  and social learning theory, 28
  and theory of reasoned action/
    planned behaviour, 34
expectancies, 27–9, 39, 43, 100, 105